MW00625337

Cambridge Pocket Clinicians provide practical, portable, note-based guidance for medical trainees, junior doctors, residents, and those from outside the field seeking an accessible overview. Written making maximum use of lists, bullet points, summary boxes, and algorithms, they allow the reader fast and ready access to essential information.

Headache

Todd J. Schwedt MD

Department of Neurology, Washington University School of Medicine, St Louis, MO, USA

Jonathan P. Gladstone MD FRCPC

Division of Neurology, Gladstone Headache Clinic, Sunnybrook Health Sciences Centre, The Hospital for Sick Children, Toronto Rehabilitation Institute and Cleveland Clinic Canada, Toronto, Ontario, Canada

R. Allan Purdy MD FRCPC

Division of Neurology, Dalhousie University, Queen Elizabeth Health Sciences Centre, Halifax, Nova Scotia, Canada

David W. Dodick MD

Department of Neurology, Mayo Clinic, Scottsdale, AZ, USA

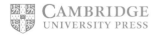
CAMBRIDGE
UNIVERSITY PRESS

Cambridge, New York, Melbourne, Madrid, Cape Town, Singapore,
São Paulo, Delhi, Dubai, Tokyo

Cambridge University Press
The Edinburgh Building, Cambridge CB2 8RU, UK

Published in the United States of America by
Cambridge University Press, New York

www.cambridge.org
Information on this title: www.cambridge.org/9780521720571

First published 2010

Printed in the United Kingdom at the University Press, Cambridge

A catalogue record for this publication is available from the British Library

Library of Congress Cataloguing in Publication data
Headache / Todd J. Schwedt ... [et al.].
    p.; cm. – (Cambridge pocket clinicians)
Includes bibliographical references and index.
ISBN 978-0-521-72057-1 (pbk.)
1. Headache – Handbooks, manuals, etc.   I. Schwedt, Todd J.   II. Series:
Cambridge pocket clinicians.
[DNLM: 1. Headache Disorders – diagnosis.   2. Emergencies.   3. Headache
Disorders – therapy.   4. Headache.   WL 342 H43151   2010]
RC392.H413 2010
616.8′491–dc22   2009050367

ISBN 978-0-521-72057-1 Paperback

Contents

Section 3 Chronic daily headaches   127

Acknowledgments

We would like to acknowledge the clinical and scientific expertise of our headache medicine friends and colleagues worldwide and thank them for teaching us so much about headache. We dedicate this small volume to those who care for patients with headache disorders.

We are grateful to the International Headache Society for permission to use the International Classification of Headache Disorders 2nd edition (ICHD-2) criteria, published in *Cephalalgia* (2004;**24** Suppl 1:9–160), throughout the book.

Preface

This new volume on headache is designed for busy clinicians who have an interest in or wish to know more about headache medicine. It is divided into three sections, mirroring the way that patients are seen in actual practice.

The first section, "Acute headaches," includes those headaches that we all need to be aware of on a daily basis, particularly in the emergency room (ER). These headache disorders can present challenges in diagnosis and treatment that are unique to emergency medicine. The second section, "Episodic headaches," is really the purview of office, clinic, and consultant practice. This section includes a variety of common, and less common but interesting, primary headache disorders. Precise diagnosis of patients with episodic headaches leads to specific directed care and good outcomes in a large number of patients. The final section, "Chronic daily headaches," encompasses some of the most complex and challenging headache disorders, many of which can consume a lot of effort and resources in order to separate out the primary from secondary disorders. The diagnosis of these patients requires expertise in headache medicine and neurology, sometimes more so than others.

The purpose of this volume is to get the reader up to speed quickly on each of the headache disorders. Each section contains highly condensed knowledge about what is important to know in terms of: key points, a general overview, clinical features, diagnosis, and treatment and outcomes. From our combined clinical knowledge of dealing daily with numerous headache patients we feel this approach will work in practice. The information learned about each headache disorder is core knowledge based on the current best evidence and experience in practice, knowledge that is unlikely to change significantly over the next few years. Each chapter ends with a short list of pertinent references for further reading, which should quickly lead the reader to the important literature, if desired. We know, however, that most busy physicians do not have the time or the inclination to do detailed reviews of the literature – nevertheless, as in all areas of clinical medicine, if the opportunity arises to study a particular headache disorder further then this book will act as an excellent guide.

Of all the headache disorders that we see on a daily basis, migraine stands out as one of the most interesting and clinically challenging disorders to diagnose and manage. You have to see hundreds of cases of migraine to get a feeling for this unique neurologic disorder because of the variations in presentation and nuances in management. On the other hand, having only seen an occasional case of cluster headache is sufficient for most clinicians to make the diagnosis with relative ease – treatment, however, being another matter!

There is an explosion of research and clinical interest in migraine and many of the new and unique primary headache disorders, and this will continue to expand in the upcoming decades as diagnosis, imaging, and therapies evolve and emerge. There is also a desire to look again at many secondary headache disorders to recognize and understand them better and to find ways to cure or lessen symptoms. Good examples of these disorders that are included in this volume are: cerebral venous sinus thrombosis, spontaneous intracranial hypotension, idiopathic intracranial hypertension, and intracranial neoplasm.

To conclude this preface, it is necessary to mention that some of the most problematic of the headache disorders are dealt with in this volume, including: medication-overuse headache, new daily persistent headache, and post-traumatic headache. There is no physician anywhere who has truly mastered the art of managing patients with these disorders, as in large part their scientific underpinnings have not been elucidated as quickly as we or others in the field of headache medicine would like. Nevertheless, as challenging as these patients can be, there is a great deal of satisfaction for the patient and their physician to work together to deal with these chronic headache disorders. This volume contains valuable information to help you practice headache medicine, a most interesting area of clinical neurology. We hope you enjoy this volume and use it regularly as a companion when you diagnose and treat your headache patients.

SECTION 1
Acute headaches

1

Introduction to the acute headaches

"Acute headaches" are those that appear suddenly. Acute headaches that are severe and reach maximal intensity within seconds to minutes are called "thunderclap headaches." Acute headaches are medical emergencies as they can be manifestations of a serious underlying abnormality such as subarachnoid hemorrhage. The potential morbidity and mortality associated with many of the causes of acute headaches makes it essential for all practitioners to be aware of the possible causes and the initial evaluation of patients presenting with an acute headache.

Patients with acute headaches often present to the emergency room for evaluation. They may have a history of a primary headache disorder such as migraine or tension-type headache. However, the acute headache stands out from the patient's usual headache. The rapid onset of a thunderclap headache and the speed by which it reaches its most severe intensity differentiate this headache type from the episodic headache. Although widely touted in traditional teaching about the headaches of subarachnoid hemorrhage, simply asking if the present headache is "the worst headache ever" is insufficient to determine if a thunderclap headache is present. Many patients who have presented emergently for evaluation of a headache will respond affirmatively to this question. However, to properly recognize a thunderclap headache the mode of onset must be considered in conjunction with headache intensity. Patients with a thunderclap headache can generally recall the moment that their headache began and can often describe this moment in vivid detail. They may liken the headache onset to "being hit in the head with a hammer" and they are frequently quite concerned about a serious underlying cause for this unusual headache.

The emergent evaluation of the patient presenting with an acute headache is initially targeted at the possibility of an underlying subarachnoid hemorrhage. The practitioner must take a quick but comprehensive history and perform physical and neurologic examinations in search of symptoms and signs suggestive of a secondary headache. The first diagnostic test should be a noncontrast computed tomography (CT) scan of the brain to look for evidence of subarachnoid blood. Since the sensitivity of CT for subarachnoid hemorrhage is less than optimal and because the risk associated with a missed diagnosis is high, lumbar puncture should be performed when brain CT is unrevealing. Evaluation by lumbar puncture should include measurement of the opening pressure and cerebrospinal fluid cell counts, protein, glucose, inspection for xanthochromia, and spectrophotometry for bilirubin when available. In patients in whom lumbar puncture evaluation is also unrevealing, evaluation of the brain with magnetic resonance imaging (MRI; with gadolinium) and evaluation of the cerebral and cervical vasculature is most often indicated in the search for other potential causes of the acute headache. A comprehensive evaluation will be negative at times, suggesting a diagnosis of "primary thunderclap headache."

In the following chapters, conditions which may present with acute headaches are discussed. Those included in Section 1 are:

- Subarachnoid hemorrhage
- Cervical artery dissection
- Acute hypertensive crisis
- Ischemic stroke

- Pituitary apoplexy
- Colloid cyst of the third ventricle
- Primary thunderclap headache
- Intracranial infection

Disorders discussed elsewhere in this text that may also occasionally present with acute headache include:

- Cerebral venous sinus thrombosis
- Spontaneous intracranial hypotension
- Complicated sinus headaches

Primary stabbing, sexual, and cough headaches may also have acute onset but tend to be episodic and are thus discussed in Section 2.

2

Subarachnoid hemorrhage

■ Key points

- Subarachnoid hemorrhage is the diagnosis of greatest urgency that must be considered in patients with the acute onset of a severe headache ("thunderclap headache")
- Up to ¼ of patients with thunderclap headache have a subarachnoid hemorrhage
- Sentinel headache, which is a thunderclap headache that precedes subarachnoid hemorrhage by days to weeks, occurs in up to 40%
- Brain CT scan is the initial evaluation, followed by cerebrospinal fluid analysis, if there is no imaging evidence of subarachnoid hemorrhage or an alternative diagnosis

■ General overview

- Subarachnoid hemorrhage most commonly presents as a severe headache of acute onset, termed "thunderclap headache"
- Patients may present with thunderclap headache in isolation, or in conjunction with other neurologic symptoms (see "Clinical features")
- Patients suspected of having subarachnoid hemorrhage must be evaluated emergently

- Rupture of an intracranial saccular aneurysm is the most common cause of subarachnoid hemorrhage; less common causes include: nonaneurysmal perimesencephalic hemorrhage, transmural arterial dissection, arteriovenous malformation, dural arteriovenous fistula, mycotic aneurysm, and cocaine use
- Although morbidity and mortality from subarachnoid hemorrhage remain high, early diagnosis and treatment is associated with improved outcomes

■ Clinical features

- Headache
  - Headache is the most common clinical manifestation of subarachnoid hemorrhage
  - Headache may occur in isolation in about one-half of patients
  - Headache is often sudden and with maximal intensity at onset or within minutes
  - Typically, the headache lasts a few days. It is atypical for the headache to last less than 2 hours
  - May be preceded by physical exertion or Valsalva
- Loss of consciousness
  - ⅓ of patients
- Seizures
  - 5%–10% of patients
- Delirium
  - 15% of patients
- Strokes
- Visual disturbances
- Nausea and vomiting
- Neck stiffness
- Photophobia

- Hunt and Hess grading system (correlates with prognosis)
    - Grade 1: Asymptomatic
    - Grade 2: Severe headache, stiff neck, no neurologic deficit except cranial nerve palsy
    - Grade 3: Drowsy, minimal neurologic deficit
    - Grade 4: Stuporous, moderate or severe hemiparesis
    - Grade 5: Deep coma, decerebrate posturing
- "Sentinel headaches"
    - These represent a premonitory warning of impending intracranial aneurysm rupture that occurs in the following days to weeks
    - Sentinel headaches occur in approximately 10%–45% of patients who have subarachnoid hemorrhage
    - Sentinel headaches are similar to those that occur with subarachnoid hemorrhage in that they begin suddenly and reach maximum intensity within seconds to minutes ("thunderclap headache")
    - Sentinel headache must be considered in the differential diagnosis of all patients who present with thunderclap headache
    - If sentinel headaches are recognized as such, appropriate intervention may allow time to intervene and avoid a catastrophic aneurysmal rupture and subarachnoid hemorrhage

■ Diagnosis (Fig. 2.1)

- Physical exam
    - Fundal hemorrhages
        - 20%–40% of patients
        - More often found in those with decreased level of consciousness
        - Detection may be difficult when photophobia is present and because of patient distress

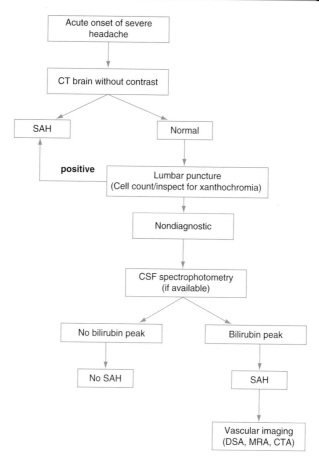

Fig. 2.1 Evaluation of suspected subarachnoid hemorrhage.
SAH, subarachnoid hemorrhage; DSA, digital subtraction angiography; MRA, magnetic resonance angiography; CTA, computed tomographic angiography.

- Meningismus
- Altered level of consciousness
- Focal neurologic deficits
- Noncontrast CT brain
  - First test in the evaluation of suspected subarachnoid hemorrhage
  - Perform as soon as possible after the onset of symptoms
    - Sensitivity nears 100% within the first 12 hours of subarachnoid hemorrhage
    - Sensitivity decreases to 50% by 1 week after hemorrhage
- Lumbar puncture
  - Perform when diagnosis is not reached by brain CT
  - Measure opening pressure, routine cell counts, and visually inspect for xanthochromia
  - Perform analysis by spectrophotometry if available
    - More sensitive after the first 12 hours – 95%
- Angiography
  - In patients with subarachnoid hemorrhage, angiography is required in search of a ruptured aneurysm
  - Conventional digital subtraction angiography (DSA) is the gold standard
  - Magnetic resonance angiography (MRA) or computed tomographic angiography (CTA) may also be used
    - MRA sensitivity ranges from 70% to 100% depending on the size of the aneurysm
      - If aneurysm is ≥6 mm, sensitivity is >95%
    - CTA sensitivity ranges from 85% to 98%

■ Treatment

- Intensive care unit
- Possible ventriculostomy for intracranial pressure monitoring

- Monitor for development of vasospasm
  - Transcranial Doppler ultrasound monitoring
  - Triple H therapy – modest hemodilution, induced hypertension, hypervolemia
  - Nimodipine
- Seizure prophylaxis with antiepileptic drugs (controversial)
- Aneurysm repair
  - Surgical clipping
  - Endovascular therapy – coiling

■ Outcome

- 10% of patients die before reaching the hospital
- There is 50% overall case fatality
- One-third of survivors have major morbidity requiring dependency for activities of daily living

■ Further reading

Edlow JA, Caplan LR. Avoiding pitfalls in the diagnosis of subarachnoid hemorrhage. *NEJM* 2000;**342**:29–36.

Hop JW, Rinkel GJ, Algra A, van Gijn J. Case-fatality rates and functional outcome after subarachnoid hemorrhage: a systematic review. *Stroke* 1997;**28**:660–664.

Koivisto T, Vanninen R, Hurskainen H, *et al.* Outcomes of early endovascular versus surgical treatment of ruptured cerebral aneurysms. A prospective randomized study. *Stroke* 2000;**31**:2369–2377.

Sidman R, Connolly E, Lemke T. Subarachnoid hemorrhage diagnosis: lumbar puncture is still needed when the computed tomography scan is normal. *Acad Emerg Med* 1996;**3**:827–831.

van Gijn J, Rinkel GJ. Subarachnoid haemorrhage: diagnosis, causes and management. *Brain* 2001;**124**(Pt 2):249–278.

3

Cervical artery dissection

■ Key points

- Dissection of the cervical internal carotid and vertebral arteries may occur after direct or indirect neck trauma, or it may occur spontaneously
- The majority of patients with cervical artery dissection have headache and about ½ have neck pain
- The majority (85%) of patients with cervical artery dissection have neurologic symptoms or signs, in addition to headache
- Many different imaging modalities may be used to diagnose cervical artery dissection including ultrasound, CT, MRI, and conventional angiography
- Evidence-based guidelines for the treatment of cervical artery dissection are not available. Treatment may include observation, antiplatelet therapy, anticoagulation, or surgical intervention

■ General overview

- Cervical artery dissection is the second most common cause of stroke in the younger (<45 years) population
- Extracranial internal carotid artery dissections are about three times more common than extracranial vertebral artery dissections
- Arterial dissections are characterized by the separation of the arterial wall layers and formation of a false lumen

- Dissection may cause significant narrowing of the arterial lumen, which may result in thrombus formation, distal embolization, and transient ischemic attack (TIA) or ischemic stroke
- Headache is the most common presenting symptom and may often precede the onset of other manifestations

■ Clinical features (Boxes 3.1 and 3.2)

- Headache
  - The most frequent presenting symptom of cervical artery dissection
  - May precede the onset of other neurologic manifestations by days or weeks
  - Frequency
    - Carotid artery dissection – 60%–95%
    - Vertebral artery dissection – 70%
  - Onset
    - Most commonly of a slow gradual onset
    - Thunderclap headache – 20%
  - Location
    - Ipsilateral to the dissected artery with carotid dissections
    - Carotid artery – frontotemporal, lower face, jaw, or ear
    - Vertebral artery – parietooccipital
  - Duration
    - Median duration of 3 days
    - When of longer duration, the majority of headaches of carotid dissections resolve within 1 week and those of vertebral dissections by 5 weeks
    - Occasionally patients have chronic headaches
- Neck pain
  - Carotid artery dissection – 25% of patients
  - Vertebral artery dissection – 50% of patients

Box 3.1 Clinical manifestations of cervical artery dissections

- Headache
- Neck pain
- Facial pain
- Horner syndrome
- Diplopia
- Amaurosis fugax
- Dysgeusia
- Pulsatile tinnitus
- Stroke

Box 3.2 Headache/facial/neck pain attributed to arterial dissection – International Headache Society diagnostic criteria

A. Any new headache, facial pain or neck pain of acute onset, with or without other neurological symptoms or signs and fulfilling criteria C and D

B. Dissection demonstrated by appropriate vascular and/or neuroimaging investigations

C. Pain develops in close temporal relation to and on the same side as the dissection

D. Pain resolves within 1 month

- Other manifestations
  - Amaurosis fugax
  - Horner syndrome – ipsilateral ptosis, miosis, anhidrosis
  - Pulsatile tinnitus (mostly ipsilateral)
  - Dysgeusia (hypoglossal nerve palsy)
  - Diplopia (oculomotor nerve palsy)
  - TIA or stroke

- Classical presentation
  - Carotid artery dissection
    - Unilateral headache
    - Horner syndrome
  - Vertebral artery dissection
    - Unilateral headache
    - Lateral medullary infarction (Wallenberg syndrome)
      - Facial and/or extremity sensory symptoms
      - Gait and/or limb ataxia
      - Dizziness/vertigo
      - Horner sign
      - Hoarseness
      - Dysphagia
      - Nystagmus
      - Nausea/vomiting
      - Diplopia

■ Diagnosis

- Physical exam
  - Neurologic exam
    - Horner syndrome – ptosis, miosis, anhidrosis
    - Lower cranial nerve palsies
    - Nystagmus
    - Ataxia – gait and/or limb
    - Sensory loss
      - Ipsilateral face and contralateral arm and leg
      - Face and/or extremities
    - Other stroke manifestations
  - Cardiovascular exam
    - Carotid and/or vertebral bruits

- Imaging
  - Imaging for cervical artery dissection may be accomplished by ultrasound, CTA, MRA, MRI of the neck using a fat saturation technique, and conventional angiography
  - Duplex ultrasound
    - Lumen tapering
    - Double lumen
    - Irregular vessel wall crossing the lumen
    - Loss of Doppler signal
  - CTA
    - Three-dimensional visualization of carotid and vertebral arteries
    - Requires contrast infusion
  - MRA
    - The procedure of choice if available
    - Tapered stenosis with extended length of arterial narrowing (Fig. 3.1)

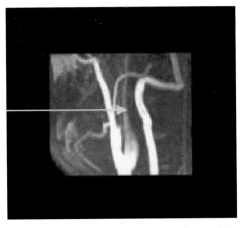

Fig. 3.1 Magnetic resonance angiogram demonstrating the tapered and narrowed lumen of the internal carotid artery, illustrative of dissection.

- MRI neck with fat saturation technique
  - "Double-lumen" sign of true and false lumen
- Conventional angiography
  - Long considered to be the gold standard for detection of dissection, however, has largely been supplanted by MRA or CTA
- MRI brain
  - Detection of cerebral infarction, which may occur secondary to dissection
  - "Crescent sign" demonstrating clot within arterial wall on T2-weighted or fluid attenuated inversion recovery (FLAIR) images (Fig. 3.2)

■ Treatment

- Asymptomatic (i.e., no ischemic cerebral symptoms)
  - Acute – antiplatelet therapy
  - Delayed diagnosis (weeks) – observation vs. antiplatelet therapy
- Symptomatic
  - Antiplatelet medication vs. anticoagulation
    - Anticoagulation may be associated with a lower rate of recurrent transient ischemic attack and stroke, but there is no controlled evidence to direct treatment to one particular antiplatelet therapy or to anticoagulation
    - Anticoagulation is associated with an increased risk of hemorrhage and thus is often avoided, especially for intracranial vertebral artery dissections because of the risk of subarachnoid hemorrhage
    - If anticoagulants are used, there is no evidence regarding duration of treatment. Some authorities use anticoagulation

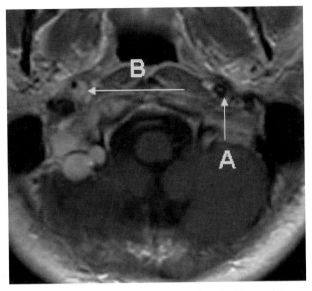

Fig. 3.2 Axial fluid attenuated inversion recovery (FLAIR) MR image of the brain demonstrating normal carotid artery flow void (*A*) and a crescent-shaped clot in the wall of the carotid artery, resulting in a small lumen (*B*).

for 3–6 months of therapy, after which antiplatelet agents may be used. Treatment decisions must be individualized

- Surgical or endovascular intervention (rarely indicated)
  - Possible indications include:
    - Aneurysmal dilatation
    - Subarachnoid hemorrhage
    - Significant arterial stenosis
    - Progressive neurologic sequelae despite medical management

■ Outcome

- Outcome chiefly depends on the presence and severity of associated stroke
- Complete or excellent recovery in about 75%
- Disabling deficits in about 20%
- Death in approximately 5%
- Intracranial dissections often have a worse prognosis
- Follow-up imaging shows normalization of the carotid artery at 3 months in the majority of patients
- Recurrent dissection in the same or another cervical artery occurs with a 1% annual incidence

■ Further reading

Dziewas R, Konrad C, Drager, *et al.* Cervical artery dissection – clinical features, risk factors, therapy and outcome in 126 patients. *J Neurol* 2003;**250**:1179–1184.

Liegeskind DS, Saver JL. Cervicocephalic arterial dissections. In: Noseworthy JH, ed. *Neurological Therapeutics Principles and Practice*. Vol 1. London: Martin Dunitz, 2003:524–535.

Lyrer P, Engelter S. Antithrombotic drugs for carotid artery dissection. *Stroke* 2004;**35**:613–614.

Silbert PL, Mokri B, Schievink WI. Headache and neck pain in spontaneous internal carotid and vertebral artery dissections. *Neurology* 1995;**45**:1517–1522.

4

Acute hypertensive crisis

■ Key points

- Abrupt elevation in blood pressure may result in the acute onset of headache
- Headache is a common symptom of hypertensive crises
- Hypertensive encephalopathy classically manifests as headache, seizures, and neurologic signs (usually visual change)
- Early diagnosis and treatment is essential to minimize the risk of permanent sequelae which may result from end-organ damage

■ General overview

- About 20% of patients with hypertensive crises report having headache
- About 25% of patients with hypertensive crises have previously undiagnosed hypertension

■ Clinical features

- Headache
  - Subacute onset is most common
  - May rarely present as a "thunderclap headache"
  - Commonly located in the posterior head (occipitonuchal)

- Moderate to severe intensity
- Throbbing
- Made worse by physical activity
- Other symptoms of hypertensive crises
  - Dizziness
  - Dyspnea
  - Chest pain
  - Psychomotor agitation
  - Epistaxis
  - Focal neurologic deficits
- Hypertensive emergency
  - Usually associated with diastolic blood pressures ≥120 mm Hg
  - Associated with end-organ damage
    - Stroke
    - Pulmonary edema
    - Encephalopathy
  - Classically presents with headache, seizures, and visual loss
  - Headache generally has an acute onset
  - Seizures are most commonly generalized tonic-clonic
  - May have associated nausea, vomiting, altered mental status, focal neurologic signs (usually visual changes such as scintillations and scotomata)
  - Papilledema and retinal hemorrhages are usually absent
  - Symptoms are usually reversible but permanent deficits may result
    - Early treatment is essential to maximize outcomes

■ Diagnosis

- The International Headache Society diagnostic criteria for headache attributed to hypertensive crisis without hypertensive encephalopathy are listed in Box 4.1

> **Box 4.1** Headache attributed to hypertensive crisis –
> International Headache Society diagnostic criteria
>
> A. Headache with at least one of the following characteristics and
>   fulfilling criteria C and D:
>   1. Bilateral
>   2. Pulsating quality
>   3. Precipitated by physical activity
> B. Hypertensive crisis defined as a paroxysmal rise in systolic (to
>   >160 mm Hg) and/or diastolic (to >120 mm Hg) blood pressure
>   but no clinical features of hypertensive encephalopathy
> C. Headache develops during hypertensive crisis
> D. Headache resolves within 1 hour after normalization of blood
>   pressure
> E. Appropriate investigations have ruled out vasopressor toxins
>   or medications as causative factors

- The International Headache Society diagnostic criteria for
  headache attributed to hypertensive encephalopathy are listed
  in Box 4.2
- Diagnosis of headache secondary to hypertension requires a
  high index of suspicion
  - Elevated blood pressure could be interpreted as a pain
    response as opposed to the underlying cause of a
    headache
- Patients presenting with thunderclap headache should
  initially be evaluated for subarachnoid hemorrhage (see
  Chapter 2)
  - Noncontrast brain CT
  - Lumbar puncture if brain CT is nondiagnostic
  - MRI brain

Box 4.2 Headache attributed to hypertensive encephalopathy – International Headache Society diagnostic criteria

A. Headache with at least one of the following characteristics and fulfilling criteria C and D:
   1. Diffuse pain
   2. Pulsating quality
   3. Aggravated by physical activity
B. Persistent blood pressure elevation to >160/100 mm Hg with at least two of the following:
   1. Confusion
   2. Reduced level of consciousness
   3. Visual disturbance (other than those of typical migraine aura) including blindness
   4. Seizures
C. Headache develops in close temporal relation to blood pressure elevation
D. Headache resolves within 3 months after effective treatment and control of hypertension
E. Other causes of the neurological symptoms have been excluded

- Posterior reversible leukoencephalopathy syndrome
  - Vasogenic edema of the white matter and cortex of the occipital, parietal, and posterior frontal lobes with potential involvement of the basal ganglia, brainstem, and cerebellum (Fig. 4.1)
  - Involvement is usually bilateral and symmetric
  - Hyperintensity on T-2 and FLAIR sequences

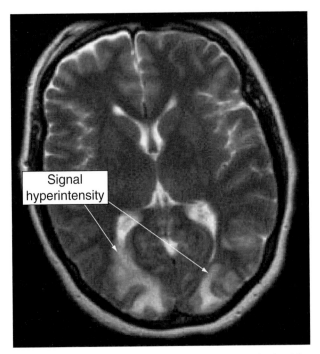

Fig. 4.1 Posterior reversible encephalopathy syndrome. T-2 weighted, axial MR image demonstrating increased signal hyperintensity in the posterior cortex and subcortical gray matter.

■ Treatment

- Blood pressure management in the acute setting
  - Goal is for at least 30%–40% reduction in systolic blood pressure
  - In hypertensive encephalopathy, mean arterial pressures should be reduced by 20%–25% within the first 1–2 hours
    - More rapid correction could exacerbate end-organ dysfunction
- Frequent blood pressure monitoring as blood pressure may be labile

■ Outcome

- The majority of patients recover completely
- A minority of patients develop cerebral infarctions or intracerebral hemorrhage

■ Further reading

Schwartz RB. Hyperperfusion encephalopathies: hypertensive encephalopathy and related conditions. *Neurologist* 2002;**8**:22–34.

Spierings ELH. Acute and chronic hypertensive headache and hypertensive encephalopathy. *Cephalalgia* 2002;**22**:313–316.

Stott VL, Hurrell MA, Anderson TJ. Reversible posterior leukoencephalopathy syndrome: a misnomer reviewed. *Intern Med J* 2005;**35**:83–90.

Tang-Wai DF, Phan TG, Wijdicks EFM. Hypertensive encephalopathy presenting with thunderclap headache. *Headache* 2001;**41**:198–200.

Zampaglione B, Pascale C, Marchisio M, Cavallo-Perin P. Hypertensive urgencies and emergencies. *Hypertension* 1996;**27**:144–147.

5

Ischemic stroke

■ Key points

- Patients with ischemic stroke may develop a headache prior to or following onset of neurologic deficits
- Headache may resemble those of a primary headache disorder or may have an acute onset
- Headache associated with ischemic stroke must be differentiated from "true migrainous infarction," which is a rare entity

■ General overview

- 25% of ischemic stroke patients have an associated headache
- Headaches are more common with:
  - Large strokes
  - Those located in the territory of the posterior circulation
    - Especially cerebellar strokes
- Headaches are less common with:
  - Transient ischemic attacks
  - Subcortical infarcts
  - Lacunar infarcts
- Risk factors for the development of headache with ischemic stroke include:
  - Younger age
  - Female gender
  - History of migraine

- Headaches occurring with ischemic stroke must be differentiated from other conditions with headache and focal neurologic deficits
  - Neoplasm
  - Reversible cerebral vasoconstriction syndromes
    - Including migrainous infarction
      - Severe cerebral hypoperfusion during migraine aura resulting in permanency of one or more of the aura symptoms due to infarct
  - Cerebral venous sinus thrombosis
  - Intracranial hemorrhage
  - Subarachnoid hemorrhage
  - Meningitis/encephalitis
  - Cerebral arteritis
  - Acute hypertensive headache

■ Clinical features

- Up to 50% of headaches associated with ischemic stroke have onset prior to neurologic deficits
- Headaches
  - Acute or subacute in onset
  - If there is a history of a primary headache disorder, the headache occurring with ischemic stroke may resemble the patient's usual headache
  - Throbbing or pressure in quality
  - Mild to moderate in intensity
- Location of headache may correlate with stroke location
  - Frontal pain is more common with anterior circulation strokes
  - Occipital pain is more common with posterior circulation strokes
  - If headache is unilateral, it is most often ipsilateral to the location of the stroke

■ Diagnosis

- Depends on:
  - Close temporal relationship between the onset of headache and signs of ischemic stroke
  - Identification of neurologic signs and/or imaging evidence for ischemic stroke
- Physical exam
  - Neurologic exam for evidence of ischemic stroke
- Tests
  - Noncontrast CT brain
  - If acute onset (thunderclap headache) and CT negative, then lumbar puncture
  - MRI brain with diffusion-weighted sequences
  - If stroke is present vascular imaging is indicated, which may be accomplished via MRA, CTA, ultrasound, or conventional angiography

■ Treatment

- Aimed at the prevention of future strokes
- Rehabilitation
- The headache may respond to many of the medications used to treat primary headache disorders
- Avoid vasoconstricting migraine medications such as the triptans and ergotamines

■ Further reading

Bousser MG, Welch KMA. Relation between migraine and stroke. *Lancet Neurol* 2005;**4**:533–542.

Ferro JM, Melo TP, Oliveira V, *et al*. A multivariate study of headache associated with ischemic stroke. *Headache* 1995;**35**:315–319.

Kumral E, Bogousslavsky J, Van Melle G, *et al*. Headache at stroke onset: the Lausanne Stroke Registry. *J Neurol Neurosurg Psychiatry* 1995;**58**:490–492.

Tentschert S, Wimmer R, Greisenegger S, *et al*. Headache at stroke onset in 2196 patients with ischemic stroke or transient ischemic attack. *Stroke* 2005;**36**:e1–e3.

Vestergaard K, Andersen G, Nillsen MI, *et al*. Headache in stroke. *Stroke* 1993;**24**:1621–1624.

6

Pituitary apoplexy

■ Key points

- Pituitary apoplexy refers to an acute clinical syndrome generally due to rapid enlargement of a pituitary adenoma from hemorrhage or infarction
- Presents with sudden-onset headache, visual impairment, vomiting, and altered cognition
- MRI of the pituitary is the imaging modality of choice
- Early identification and treatment may result in improved outcomes

■ General overview

- Pituitary apoplexy is rare but potentially lethal
  - 0.6%–9% of treated pituitary adenomas
  - More frequent in males than females (~2:1)
  - Mean age in the fifth decade
- It refers to an acute-onset clinical syndrome that is most commonly due to rapid enlargement of a pituitary adenoma from hemorrhage, infarction, or hemorrhagic infarction
  - Most commonly occurs in patients with undiagnosed pituitary tumors
    - Nonfunctioning or hyperfunctional tumors
  - May occur in the normal pituitary gland
- Arterial hypertension may be a predisposing factor

■ Clinical features

- Acute onset of headache, vomiting, visual disturbance, ophthalmoplegia, and altered consciousness
  - Headache
  - Most common presenting symptom
    - Reported by about 90% of patients
  - Thunderclap headache
    - Sudden onset
    - Severe intensity
  - Frequently retroorbital in location
- Nausea/vomiting
  - Up to 80% of patients
- Meningismus
- Visual change
  - Decreased visual acuity
    - Including blindness
  - Visual field deficits
- Ophthalmoplegia
  - Cranial nerve III palsy most common
  - Cranial nerve VI or IV palsy less common
- Altered consciousness
  - Confusion
  - Decreased level of consciousness
- Acute adrenal insufficiency
  - Acute hypotension
  - Cardiovascular collapse

■ Diagnosis

- Laboratory
  - Hypopituitarism in the majority

- Manifests as deficiency of one or more:
  - Gonadotrophins (follicle-stimulating hormone, luteinizing hormone)
  - Testosterone
  - Cortisol
  - Insulin-like growth factor
  - Thyrotrophin
  - Prolactin
  - A minority of patients have elevated white blood cell counts and/or hyponatremia
- Imaging
  - Skull radiograph
    - Enlarged sella
  - Brain CT is inadequate
    - Low sensitivity
    - Diagnostic in ¼ of cases or less
  - Contrast and noncontrast brain MRI
    - Test of choice
    - Higher sensitivity for detection of pituitary tumor, necrosis, and hemorrhage

■ Treatment

- Conservative therapy
  - Includes fluid and electrolyte balance and replacement of deficient hormones
  - Can be associated with recurrent apoplexy
- Corticosteroid replacement
  - Initiated as soon as pituitary apoplexy is suspected
- Fluid and electrolyte balance
- Surgical treatment

  - May be indicated when there is diminished level of consciousness, hypothalamic disturbance, or visual impairment
  - Emergent surgery may be indicated when there is progressive worsening of vision, sudden onset of blindness, or diminished level of consciousness
  - Early surgery (first week) may be indicated if there is visual impairment
- Radiation therapy
  - May be necessary if there is tumor recurrence

■ Outcome

- Up to 90% of patients have a good recovery
  - Majority of associated neurologic deficits return to normal
    - Visual deficits and oculomotor pareses improve in the majority
    - Early treatment (within the first week) may be associated with greater recovery
- Most require long-term pituitary hormone replacement

■ Further reading

Dubuisson AS, Beckers A, Stevenaert A. Classical pituitary tumour apoplexy: clinical features, management and outcomes in a series of 24 patients. *Clin Neurol Neurosurg* 2007;**109**:63–70.

Freeman WD, Maramattom B, Czervionke L, Manna EM. Pituitary apoplexy. *Neurocrit Care* 2005;**3**:174–176.

Randeva HS, Schoebel J, Byrne J, *et al.* Classical pituitary apoplexy: clinical features, management and outcome. *Clin Endocrinol* 1999;**51**:181–188.

Semple, PL, Webb MK, de Villiers JC, Laws ER. Pituitary apoplexy. *Neurosurgery* 2005;**56**:65–73.

Sibal L, Ball SG, Connolly V, *et al.* Pituitary apoplexy: a review of clinical presentation, management and outcome in 45 cases. *Pituitary* 2004;**7**:157–163.

7

Colloid cyst of the third ventricle

■ Key points

- Colloid cysts are benign tumors that are most commonly located in the third ventricle near the foramen of Monro
- Hydrocephalus may develop if a cyst blocks cerebrospinal fluid flow
- Acute hydrocephalus may result in headache, loss of consciousness, cognitive changes, seizures, coma, and death
- Brain MRI is the diagnostic test of choice
- Treatment may consist of observation, aspiration, microsurgical resection, or endoscopic resection

■ General overview

- Colloid cysts are benign tumors that constitute about 0.5%–1% of all intracranial tumors
- Commonly attached by a "stalk" to the anterior superior aspect of the third ventricle
- Most often found in patients between 30 and 60 years of age
- Intermittent obstruction of cerebrospinal fluid flow may result in acute hydrocephalus and symptoms ranging from mild headache to death
- The size of the cyst varies widely and is not helpful in predicting symptoms or outcome

■ Clinical features

- Headache
- Most common symptom
  - Typically bifrontal or generalized
  - Severe in intensity
  - Throbbing or aching
  - Typically begins and stops abruptly
  - Endures for hours to days
  - Initiation, relief or change in intensity of headache with head movements and/or changes in posture
- Visual changes
- Vomiting
- Vertigo
- Ataxia
- Short-term memory deficits
- Urinary incontinence
- Seizures
- Drop attacks/syncope
- Coma
- Death
  - Sudden death often occurring within the first week of symptom onset

■ Diagnosis

- Physical exam
  - Papilledema present in the majority
  - Examination is completely normal in a minority
- CT brain (Fig. 7.1)
  - May miss the diagnosis in up to ⅓ of cases
    - Due to a cyst that is isodense to brain tissue

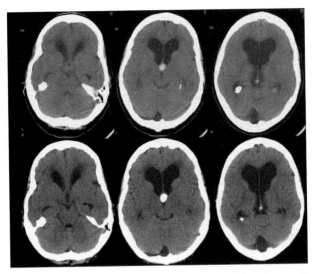

Fig. 7.1 Transverse CT view of colloid cyst with some ventricular enlargement over time.

- Hyperdense to brain tissue in the majority
- Round or oval mass varying in size from 3 mm to 40 mm
- Thin rim of enhancement with contrast administration
- Ventriculomegaly
- MRI brain (Fig. 7.2)
  - Imaging test of choice
  - Cyst has heterogeneous intensity
  - Most are hyperintense on T1-weighted images and hypointense on T2-weighted images
  - Ventriculomegaly

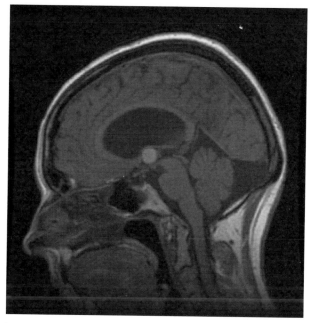

Fig. 7.2 Sagittal MR view of a colloid cyst of the third ventricle with secondary hydrocephalus.

■ Treatment

- Conservative therapy
  - Could be considered in some patients:
    - Asymptomatic
    - No neuroimaging progression
    - Older age
- Observation
  - Serial neuroimaging

- Microsurgical resection
  - Gold standard treatment
  - May be associated with relatively high operative morbidity and mortality
- Aspiration
  - Cyst wall remains
    - Associated with a high recurrence rate
  - Endoscopic resection
    - Alternative to microsurgical resection
    - May be associated with shorter operative, hospitalization, and rehabilitation time
    - May be associated with fewer surgical complications
    - Experience thus far is inconclusive regarding long-term outcome and cyst recurrence

■ Further reading

Armao D, Castillo M, Chen H, Kwock L. Colloid cyst of the third ventricle: imaging-pathologic correlation. *Am J Neuroradiol* 2000;**21**:1470–1477.

Desai KI, Nadkarni TD, Muzumdar DP, Goel AH. Surgical management of colloid cyst of the third ventricle – a study of 105 cases. *Surg Neurol* 2002;**57**:295–304.

Hellwig D, Bauer BL, Schulte M, Gatscher S, *et al.* Neuroendoscopic treatment for colloid cysts of the third ventricle: the experience of a decade. *Neurosurgery* 2003;**52**:525–533.

Pollock BE, Schreiner SA, Huston J. A theory on the natural history of colloid cysts of the third ventricle. *Neurosurgery* 2000;**46**:1077–1083.

Young WB, Silberstein SD. Paroxysmal headache caused by colloid cyst of the third ventricle: case report and review of the literature. *Headache* 1997;**37**:15–20.

8

Primary thunderclap headache

■ Key points

- "Thunderclap headache" refers to a severe headache with sudden onset that reaches maximum intensity in less than 1 minute
- Thunderclap headache is considered a medical emergency
- A variety of secondary causes may present with thunderclap headache and a normal neurologic examination. Some may elude detection on initial CT head and cerebrospinal fluid examination
- Reversible cerebral vasoconstriction (Fig. 8.1) may be present in up to 60% of patients with nonhemorrhagic thunderclap headache and requires cerebrovascular imaging for detection (MRA, CTA, angiography)
- Primary thunderclap headache is a diagnosis of exclusion
  - The multiple causes of thunderclap headache, including subarachnoid hemorrhage, must be excluded prior to assigning a "primary" diagnosis

■ General overview

- Onset of pain is likened to being hit by a "clap of thunder"
- Thunderclap headache may be secondary to an underlying cause or may be idiopathic

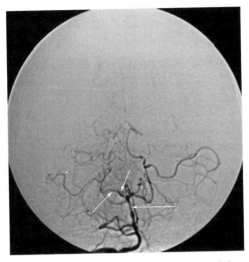

Fig. 8.1 Angiogram illustrating multiple areas of vasoconstriction and vasodilatation, typical of reversible cerebral vasoconstriction syndrome.

- There are multiple causes of thunderclap headache (Box 8.1)
- If a comprehensive evaluation for causes of secondary thunderclap headache is unrevealing, "primary thunderclap headache" may be the diagnosis

■ Clinical features

- Headache
  - Sudden in onset
    - Patients can generally recall the exact moment when the headache began
  - Severe

Box 8.1 Causes of thunderclap headache

- Subarachnoid hemorrhage
- Sentinel headache (warning headache that occurs prior to subarachnoid hemorrhage)
- Cervical artery dissection (internal carotid or vertebral artery)
- Cerebral venous sinus thrombosis
- Spontaneous intracranial hypotension (spontaneous cerebrospinal fluid leak)
- Acute hypertensive crisis
- Pituitary apoplexy
- Retroclival hematoma
- Complicated sinusitis
- Ischemic stroke
- Reversible cerebral vasoconstriction syndrome
- Third ventricular colloid cyst
- Intracranial infection

- Reaches maximum intensity in <1 minute
- Location is variable, but often posterior
- Duration ranging from 1 hour to weeks
- Primary thunderclap headache should not be associated with fever, alteration in consciousness, altered cognition, or focal neurologic deficits
  - Presence of associated abnormalities suggests "secondary thunderclap headache"

■ Diagnosis

- The International Headache Society diagnostic criteria for "primary thunderclap headache" are listed in Box 8.2

> **Box 8.2 Primary thunderclap headache – International Headache Society diagnostic criteria**
>
> A. Severe head pain fulfilling criteria B and C
> B. Both of the following characteristics:
>   1. Sudden onset, reaching maximum intensity in <1 minute
>   2. Endures from 1 hour to 10 days
> C. Does not recur regularly over subsequent weeks or months
> D. Not attributed to another disorder (normal cerebrospinal fluid and normal brain imaging are needed)

- The diagnosis of primary thunderclap headache can only be made after a comprehensive evaluation for potential causes
  - Physical examination
    - Normal
    - No evidence of fever, acute hypertension, meningismus, acute fundoscopic abnormalities, neurologic deficits
  - Noncontrast CT brain
    - No acute abnormality
      - No evidence of subarachnoid hemorrhage
  - Lumbar puncture
    - Normal opening pressure and cerebrospinal fluid evaluation
      - Includes protein, glucose, cell counts, visual inspection, and spectrophotometry (if available)
  - MRI brain with and without gadolinium
    - No identified cause of headache
    - No pachymeningeal enhancement or cerebellar tonsillar descent
    - No ischemic or hemorrhagic stroke

- No pituitary apoplexy
- No colloid cyst
- No posterior leukoencephalopathy
- No retroclival hematoma
  - Vascular imaging
    - MRA, CTA, or conventional catheter angiography
      - No evidence of aneurysm
      - No evidence of arterial dissection
      - No evidence of cerebral vasoconstriction
    - Venography
      - No evidence of cerebral venous sinus thrombosis

■ Treatment

- No specific treatment indicated
- Analgesics for pain

■ Outcome

- Benign prognosis
- Does not recur regularly over subsequent weeks or months
  - Can recur within the first week after onset

■ Further reading

Calabrese LH, Dodick DW, Schwedt TJ, Singhal AB. Narrative review: reversible cerebral vasoconstriction syndromes. *Ann Intern Med* 2007;**146**:34–44.

Ducros A, Boukobza M, Porcher R, *et al.* The clinical and radiological spectrum of reversible cerebral vasoconstriction syndrome. A prospective series of 67 patients. *Brain* 2007;**130**:3091–3101.

Markus HS. A prospective follow up of thunderclap headache mimicking subarachnoid hemorrhage. *J Neurol Neurosurg Psychiatry* 1991;**54**:1117–1118.

Schwedt TJ, Matharu MS, Dodick DW. Thunderclap headache. *Lancet Neurol* 2006;**5**:621–631.

Widjicks EFM, Kerkhoff H, Van Gijn J. Long-term follow-up of 71 patients with thunderclap headache mimicking subarachnoid haemorrhage. *Lancet* 1988;**2**:68–70.

9

Intracranial infection

■ Key points

- Headaches may occur secondary to meningitis, encephalitis, and intracranial abscess
- Although headaches are common in patients with central nervous system infections, they are rarely the only clinical manifestation
- The possibility of an underlying infectious etiology must be considered in all patients with new, daily, persistent headache
- Diagnosis is based on history, physical exam, laboratory evaluation, imaging, and/or cerebrospinal fluid analysis

■ General overview

- Headaches are a common manifestation of intracranial infections such as meningitis, encephalitis, and abscess
- In addition to headache, patients with intracranial infections usually have other symptoms and signs suggestive of infection
- Headache may be the sole manifestation of indolent infections such as fungal meningitis or aseptic meningitis
  - More common in immunosuppressed patients
- Occasionally, intracranial infections can present with acute headaches ("thunderclap headaches")
  - More commonly of subacute onset

■ Clinical features

- Intracranial infections most commonly present with a constellation of four symptoms: headache, fever, nuchal rigidity, ± mental status change
  - Full tetrad present in only a minority of patients
- Typical clinical symptoms may be absent with indolent infections and in immunosuppressed patients
- Headache
  - May be the first symptom of intracranial infection
  - Headache features are nonspecific
    - May resemble common primary headache disorders such as tension-type headache and migraine headache
  - Acute or subacute onset
  - Severe
  - Holocephalic
  - May be progressive in nature
- Nuchal rigidity
- Nausea/vomiting
- Photophobia
- Back pain
- Fever/chills
- Focal neurologic deficits
- Altered mentation
  - Drowsiness
  - Delirium
  - Stupor
  - Coma
- Malaise
- Seizures

■ Diagnosis

- Physical exam
  - Vital signs
  - Level of consciousness
  - Level of cognition
  - Funduscopic examination for evidence of papilledema
  - Focal neurologic deficits
  - Meningismus
    - Kernig sign
      - Pain caused by flexing the patient's hip to 90° and then extending the patient's knee
    - Brudzinski sign
      - Forward flexion of the patient's neck causes flexion of the patient's hips and knees
- Blood tests
  - Leukocytosis
  - Elevated acute inflammatory markers
- Brain CT
  - If there is any concern over the possibility of increased intracranial pressure, brain CT is performed prior to lumbar puncture
- Lumbar puncture
  - Cerebrospinal fluid analysis is the mainstay of diagnosis
  - Pattern of results depends on the specific underlying disease process
  - Elevated white blood cell count
  - Increased protein
  - Glucose normal to low depending on underlying process
  - Opening pressure may be elevated
  - Depending on the clinical scenario, specific testing for viruses, bacteria, fungi, and acid-fast bacilli may be indicated

■ Treatment

- Treatment of the underlying meningitis, encephalitis, or abscess
- Analgesics for headache
- Antipyretics

■ Further reading

Lamonte M, Silberstein SD, Marcelis JF. Headache associated with aseptic meningitis. *Headache* 1995;**35**:520–526.

Pizon AF, Bonner MR, Wang HE, Kaplan RM. Ten years of clinical experience with adult meningitis at an urban academic medical center. *J Emerg Med* 2006;**30**:367–370.

Rashmi K. Aseptic meningitis: diagnosis and management. *Indian J Pediatr* 2005;**72**:57–63.

Scelsa SN, Lipton RB, Sander H, Herskovitz S. Headache characteristics in hospitalized patients with Lyme disease. *Headache* 1995;**35**:125–130.

SECTION 2
Episodic headaches

10

Introduction to the episodic headaches

Headache is the most common symptom that humans experience. The vast majority of individuals experience a headache at some point during their lifetime. The most common pattern of headache in the general population is episodic or intermittent headaches. Individuals with "episodic headaches" may get headaches once a year, once a month or several times per week. The headaches typically wax and wane in frequency over time. When headaches occur on more days than not (i.e., >15 days per month), this is considered to be "chronic daily headache," and this pattern of headache disorders will be discussed in the third section of this book.

The overwhelming majority of individuals with episodic headaches have a benign primary headache disorder – it is uncommon for secondary or sinister causes of headache to present with long-standing episodic headaches. The most common secondary causes of episodic headache include:

- Headaches induced by acute substance use (i.e., due to use of certain medications such as sildenafil) or substance withdrawal (i.e., alcohol hangover headache)
- Headaches attributable to eyestrain (i.e., refractive errors)
- Headaches attributable to sinus infections (although this is rarely a cause of frequent (>1/month) headaches)

> **Box 10.1** Historical features that should raise concern of a secondary cause for headache. The physician must *"SNOOP 4"* these red flags in the history of every patient presenting for the first time with headache
>
> - *S*ystemic symptoms (fever, weight loss) or *S*ystemic disease (malignancy)
> - *N*eurologic symptoms or signs (cognition, visual, focal)
> - *O*nset sudden (acute or thunderclap headache)
> - *O*nset after age 50 years
> - *P*revious headache history (new or different)
> - *P*ersistent (daily) and/or *P*rogressive
> - *P*recipitation by Valsalva (cough, bending)
> - *P*ostural

- Headaches due to cold-stimulus (also called as "ice-cream" headache)
- And less commonly – headaches attributable to intermittent medical problems (i.e. cardiac cephalalgia) or procedures (i.e. dialysis headache)

In the absence of any "red flags" suggestive of a secondary cause (see Box 10.1), the physician's task is to identify the correct primary headache disorder in order to guide rational treatment. In this section we highlight the four categories of primary episodic headache disorders. The following headache types will be reviewed:

- Migraine
  - Migraine without and with aura
  - Migraine variants – hemiplegic migraine and basilar-type migraine
- Episodic tension-type headache

- Trigeminal autonomic cephalalgias
  - Cluster headache
  - Paroxysmal hemicrania
  - SUNCT syndrome
- Other primary headache syndromes
  - Hypnic headache
  - Primary stabbing headache
  - Primary cough headache
  - Primary sexual headache

While episodic tension-type headache (ETTH) is the most common headache type in the general population, due to its mild intensity, ETTH does not commonly prompt an individual to consult their physician specifically about their headaches. By contrast, owing to its severity and functional disability, migraine is overwhelming the most common headache type presenting to physicians in primary care, walk-in clinics, and emergency room settings. Cluster headache is uncommon; however, it is an extremely important headache type not to overlook. Unfortunately, the average cluster headache patient goes 6 years from the time of symptom presentation until the correct diagnosis of cluster headache is made.

Migraine, tension-type headache, and cluster headache can also be chronic conditions. Chronic migraine, chronic tension-type headache, and chronic cluster are discussed separately in Section 3.

11

Episodic migraine headache

■ Key points

- Migraine is the most common type of headache leading to family physician, neurologist and emergency room visits
- Most episodic, recurring, "bad" headaches are migraine
- Migraine is considered by the World Health Organization to be one of the top 20 most disabling conditions
- Effective migraine management includes migraine education, lifestyle modifications (to minimize migraine triggers), and abortive medications for acute attacks. In some patients, nonpharmacologic treatment modalities (biofeedback, relaxation training, cognitive-behavioral therapy) or pharmacologic prophylactic treatment (i.e., tricyclic antidepressants, β-blockers, anticonvulsants, calcium-channel blockers, etc.) are necessary to minimize attacks

■ General overview

- Episodic migraine headache is a common headache disorder affecting approximately 18% of women and 6% of men
- Migraine often begins is childhood or adolescence, but it is most prevalent between the ages of 20 and 45
- The average migraineur has approximately two migraines per month

- Migraines may begin at any time of the day or night. It is not uncommon for a migraine to wake an individual from sleep or for the migraineur to wake up in the morning with a fully developed migraine

■ Clinical features

- Headache
  - Last from 4 to 72 hours (1–72 hours in children) untreated; approximately 50% of migraines last at least 24 hours
  - Unilateral in approximately ⅔ of individuals; usually fluctuates between sides but is occasionally "side-locked" (always involving the same side)
  - Pulsating or throbbing in approximately 75%
  - Typically moderate to severe in intensity
  - Usually fronto-temporal but can be retro-orbital, parietal, occipito-nuchal, or mid-facial
  - Typically aggravated by physical activity/exertion/straining and/or causes avoidance of physical activity/exertion/straining
- Associated features
  - Nausea occurs during some attacks in about ⅔ of patients
  - Vomiting in approximately 20% of migraineurs; however, vomiting does not typically occur with each attack. Vomiting is more common in childhood and adolescent migraine than in adult migraine
  - Photophobia (heightened sensitivity to light) and phonophobia (heightened sensitivity to sound) are common
  - Osmophobia (heightened sensitivity to odors) is also common during a migraine attack. Strong perfumes, colognes, or cooking smells are often unusually disagreeable

- Dizziness, light-headedness, or vertigo may occur. Due to kinesiophobia (heightened sensitivity to movement) and exacerbation of headache intensity with physical activity/straining, most migraineurs prefer to lie down or be still during an attack
- Lethargy or an irresistible desire to sleep is common
- Cognitive changes, including a reduced ability to concentrate and difficulty with abstract thought or memory, can occur
- Changes in mood, including irritability or depressed mood, may occur
- Cranial autonomic symptoms including mild ptosis, conjunctival injection, lacrimation, nasal congestion or rhinorrhea can occur. These symptoms are not specific to cluster headache

- Aura
  - Transient focal neurologic symptom(s) that precedes (or coincides) with the migraine headache. Occasionally, the aura can occur on its own without an accompanying headache (typical migraine aura without headache, previously referred to as "acephalgic migraine", "late-life migraine accompaniments", or "migraine equivalents")
  - Auras are present in approximately 20% of patients with episodic migraine (this is referred to as migraine with aura – previously called "classical migraine")
  - Auras are fully reversible and usually last for 5–60 minutes
  - The most common form of aura is visual; sensory auras are second most common and speech auras are infrequent
  - If more than one aura type is involved, the symptoms typically progress sequentially from one aura type to the next

- Visual auras consist of fully reversible visual symptoms including positive features (e.g., flickering lights, spots, scintillating scotomas) or negative features (i.e., blurriness or loss of vision in a hemifield)
- Sensory auras consist of fully reversible hemisensory symptoms including positive features (i.e., pins and needles) and/or negative features (i.e., numbness). Typically, sensory auras are cheiro-oral (sequential progression from the fingertips to the lips)
- Speech auras consist of fully reversible dysphasic speech disturbances (i.e., word-finding errors, semantic or phonemic paraphasias)
- Motor auras (unilateral weakness or hemiplegia) are specific for a unique migraine variant called hemiplegic migraine (sporadic or familial)
- Prodrome
  - Premonitory symptoms occur in many migraine patients and aid the individual (and/or their family members) in predicting a forthcoming migraine
  - Changes in mood or behavior (irritability, depression, apathy, euphoria)
  - Neurologic symptoms (difficulty thinking or concentrating; neck pain or tightness)
  - Fatigue symptoms (excessive tiredness or yawning)
  - Alimentary symptoms (hunger, food cravings, anorexia, nausea)
- Postdrome
  - Following the resolution of the headache phase of the migraine, some migraineurs feel fatigued, weak, listless, or lethargic; conversely, some feel refreshed or even euphoric

■ Triggers

- Change in sleep routine (sleep deprivation, sleeping in)
- Delayed or skipped meals, especially breakfast or lunch
- Acute stress or let-down from stress (i.e., after an exam or assignment, end of the work week, first day of vacation)
- Change in weather patterns (barometric pressure changes)
- Certain foods (i.e., red wine, chocolate, aged cheeses, monosodium glutamate, aspartame, processed meats)
- Change in hormone levels (menstruation or ovulation)
- Caffeine withdrawal

■ Diagnosis

- The diagnosis of migraine is based on operational diagnostic criteria (Box 11.1)
- The differential diagnosis of episodic migraine includes episodic tension-type headache (see Chapter 14), cluster headache (see Chapter 15), and chronic migraine (see Chapter 25)
- The main differences between tension-type headache and migraine are that tension-type headache is of lower severity (mild to moderate), more likely to be bilateral, lacks a throbbing quality, is not affected by exertion, lacks prominent gastrointestinal symptoms (nausea, vomiting), and is associated with significantly less headache-related disability
- The main differences between cluster headache and migraine are that cluster headache attacks are shorter in duration (15–180 minutes), more frequent (up to several times daily), exclusively unilateral, associated with motor agitation, and are associated with more prominent cranial autonomic symptoms (ptosis, lacrimation, conjunctival injection)

Box 11.1 Episodic migraine without aura – International Headache Society diagnostic criteria

Diagnostic criteria:

A. At least 5 attacks fulfilling criteria B–D
B. Headache attacks lasting 4–72 hours (untreated or unsuccessfully treated)
C. Headache has at least two of the following characteristics:
   1. unilateral location
   2. pulsating quality
   3. moderate or severe pain intensity
   4. aggravation by or causing avoidance of routine physical activity (*eg*, walking or climbing stairs)
D. During headache at least one of the following:
   1. nausea and/or vomiting
   2. photophobia and phonophobia
E. Not attributed to another disorder

- Episodic migraine is a clinical diagnosis and should be based upon a thorough clinical history and a normal general and neurologic exam
- The American Academy of Neurology together with the US Headache Consortium developed guidelines for neuroimaging in migraine patients. Patients with stable episodic migraine who have not experienced a recent change in headache pattern, seizures, and have a normal neurologic examination do not require diagnostic investigations (serology, neuroimaging, electroencephalogram (EEG), or lumbar puncture)
- Neuroimaging (computed tomography (CT) or MRI depending on the diagnosis being considered) is recommended if any "red flags" are identified on history or physical exam (see Chapter 10).

- EEG in episodic headache should be restricted to patients with symptoms suggestive of a seizure such as loss of consciousness
- US Headache Consortium performed a meta-analysis of studies evaluating neuroimaging for the work-up of episodic migraine with normal neurologic examination and found the rate of significant intracranial abnormalities to be 0.2% (with an upper 95% confidence limit of 0.6%) – this is comparable to the frequency of abnormalities in asymptomatic, healthy volunteers

■ Treatment

- Treatment of migraine headache includes lifestyle modifications to minimize headache occurrence, non-pharmacologic treatment modalities and acute and prophylactic pharmacologic treatment
- An important early step in management is migraine-specific education about trigger factors and implementation of lifestyle modifications to avoid/minimize trigger factors
- Acute migraines are typically managed by over-the-counter (OTC) and/or prescription medications. All acute therapies are more effective when taken earlier in the migraine attack when the pain is milder
- OTC analgesics
  - Effective OTC analgesics include acetylsalicylic acid, NSAIDs, and acetaminophen. Combination products with caffeine are also effective
- Prescription acute migraine options:
  - Prescription-strength NSAIDs
  - Codeine-containing analgesics

- Butalbital-containing analgesics
- Ergotamines (oral, rectal suppository, or intranasal)
- Opioids
- Triptans (oral tablet, oral disintegrating tablet, intranasal, or subcutaneous)
  - Triptans are the most efficacious class of medications available for migraine
  - There are seven different brands of triptans available in the United States and several different formulations
  - The triptans are more similar than they are different; however, there are individual differences between the triptans and the triptan formulations that can lead to individual response differences
  - Triptans are effective (decrease the pain from moderate/severe to mild or no pain) in approximately two out of three attacks in ⅔ of individuals
  - Triptans should be avoided in individuals with cardiovascular or cerebrovascular disease, peripheral vascular disease, Prinzmetal angina, and hemiplegic or basilar migraine
- Antiemetics
  - Antiemetics (diphenhydramine, metoclopramide, chlorpromazine) are useful adjunctive therapies to minimize migraine-related nausea and vomiting
- Prophylactic therapy
  - May be considered when headaches are frequent (≥3–4 per month), disabling (missed work, school or diminished quality of life), the cost of acute migraine management is prohibitive, or acute migraine medications are contraindicated, ineffective, or poorly tolerated

- The goal of prophylactic therapy is to decrease headache frequency, severity, duration and acute migraine medication requirements
- Prophylactic therapies include tricyclic antidepressants (amitriptyline, nortriptyline), β-blockers (propranolol, atenolol, metoprolol, nadolol), anti-convulsants (topiramate, valproic acid, gabapentin), calcium-channel blockers (verapamil, flunarizine), and serotonergic agents (methysergide)
- There is modest evidence to support the use of various naturopathic/herbal remedies including feverfew (*Tanacetum parthenium*), riboflavin (vitamin B_2), magnesium, butterbur (*Petasites* hybrid), and coenzyme Q10
- Nonpharmacologic therapy
  - There is sufficient evidence to support the use of relaxation training, thermal or electromyographic biofeedback, and cognitive–behavioral therapy in migraine management
  - At this time, there is insufficient evidence to support the use of acupuncture, chiropractic manipulation, cranial-sacral therapy, detoxification therapies, hypnosis, occlusal adjustment, osteopathic manipulation, and transcutaneous electrical stimulation

■ Outcome

- Migraine typically begins during childhood, adolescence or young adulthood
- Approximately 90% of migraineurs develop their first migraine by age 45
- Migraine typically becomes less frequent, less severe, and is associated with less prominent gastrointestinal symptoms by age 50 in men or by menopause in women
- Approximately 10% of individuals with episodic migraine develop chronic migraine

■ Further reading

Dodick D, Lipton RB, Martin V, *et al*. Consensus statement: cardiovascular safety profile of triptans (5-HT agonists) in the acute treatment of migraine. *Headache* 2004;**44**:414–425.

Frishberg BM, Rosenberg JH, Matchar DB, *et al*. Evidence-based guidelines in the primary care setting: neuroimaging in patients with nonacute headache. Available at: http://www.aan.com/public/practiceguidelines.

Gladstone JP, Dodick DW. Acute migraine – which triptan? *Pract Neurol* 2004;**4**:6–19.

Gladstone JP, Eross EJ, Dodick DW. Migraine in special populations. Treatment strategies for children and adolescents, pregnant women, and the elderly. *Postgrad Med* 2004;**115**:39–50.

Goadsby PJ. Migraine pathophysiology. *Headache* 2006;**45**(Suppl 1):S14–S24.

Lewis D, Ashwal S, Hershey A, *et al*. Practice parameter: pharmacological treatment of migraine headache in children and adolescents: report of the American Academy of Neurology Quality Standards Subcommittee and the Practice Committee of the Child Neurology Society. *Neurology* 2004;**63**:2215–2224.

Lipton RB, Bigal ME, Goadsby PJ. Double-blind clinical trials of oral triptans vs other classes of acute migraine medication – a review. *Cephalalgia* 2004;**24**:321–332.

Silberstein SD. Practice parameter: Evidence-based guidelines for migraine headache (an evidence-based review). *Neurology* 2000;**55**:754–762.

12

Hemiplegic migraine

■ Key points

- Hemiplegic migraine is a rare subtype of migraine with aura
- There are two subtypes of hemiplegic migraine: familial and sporadic
- Aura consists of reversible unilateral weakness/hemiplegia plus one or more of reversible sensory, visual, or language symptoms
- Aura symptoms can last from a few minutes to a few hours or days
- Three different genetic abnormalities have been identified: familial hemiplegic migraine types 1, 2, and 3 (FHM 1, FHM2, FHM3). Each mutation leads to an alteration in ionic conduction across the neuronal or glial cell membrane, altered membrane potential, and reduced threshold for depolarization (hyperexcitability)
- There is no proven effective treatment for hemiplegic migraine; analgesics are the treatment of choice for acute attacks and verapamil, acetazolamide, or anticonvulsants (topiramate or divalproex sodium) may be tried for prophylaxis

■ General overview

- Hemiplegic migraine is rare, with population estimates ranging from 1:20 000 to 1:50 000
- Familial hemiplegic migraine is thought to be more common than sporadic hemiplegic migraine

- Males and females are equally affected in familial hemiplegic migraine whereas in sporadic hemiplegic migraine there is a 2–4:1 female to male ratio
- Mean age of onset is between 12 and 18 years
- 95% have their first attack by age 45
- By age 50, attacks typically stop or evolve into typical migraine aura with headache (also termed "classical migraine") or typical aura without headache
- Frequency of attacks ranges from a few per week to only a few throughout life (mean 3–4 attacks per year)

■ Clinical features

- Headache
  - Overall, share the same characteristics with migraine with or without aura
  - Duration from several hours to several days (mean 24 hours)
  - Unilateral (may alternate sides) or bilateral
- Aura symptoms and signs
  - Auras consist of weakness/hemiplegia plus one or more of reversible visual, sensory or speech symptoms
  - Aura symptoms progress over 15–30 minutes and may last from several hours to several days. Rare cases of symptoms and signs lasting up to months have been reported
  - Motor aura (i.e., weakness or hemiparesis) is the characteristic feature of hemiplegic migraine. Hemiplegic migraine is the only migraine subtype that includes weakness as an aura symptom
  - In typical migraine with aura (also termed classical migraine) visual aura is the most common aura subtype, followed by sensory auras; speech auras are a distant third in frequency.

    In addition to hemiplegia, in hemiplegic migraine, sensory auras are the most frequent aura subtype followed closely by visual and speech auras

- The aura usually begins with progressive visual or sensory symptoms; motor and language symptoms are infrequently the initial symptom
- Language symptoms may occur independent of the affected side (motor, speech, or visual symptoms)
- Basilar-type migraine symptoms have been noted in up to 75% of hemiplegic migraine patients
- Auras are often prolonged; >50% last >1 hour (unlike typical aura with migraine where most auras last <60 minutes)
- Note that the aura symptoms may switch sides between attacks
- Unilateral weakness or paralysis may be noted on examination
- Unilateral hyper-reflexia and/or positive Babinski response may be noted
- Decreased speech fluency, paraphasias may be observed
- Cerebellar features
  - Up to 20% of individuals with FHM1 have cerebellar symptoms; cerebellar symptoms are uncommon in the other familial hemiplegic migraine subtypes
  - In FHM1, subclinical cerebellar findings may be noted on examination, including nystagmus, gait or limb ataxia, and dysarthria
  - In FHM1, vermian (midline cerebellar) or generalized atrophy may be noted on magnetic resonance imaging (MRI)
  - Cerebellar symptoms may cause some disability; however, rarely are patients wheelchair bound or requiring assisted devices
- More severe attacks
  - Consist of impaired/decreased level of consciousness ranging from confusion to coma, fever, meningismus, and seizures

- Often occur in children or young adults and may be triggered by mild head trauma
- Recovery is usually complete and may take days or weeks
- Trigger factors
  - Stress
  - Head trauma
  - Other common migraine triggers (dietary, weather, menstruation) are infrequently reported

■ Diagnosis

- The diagnosis of familial or sporadic hemiplegic migraine is based on operational diagnostic criteria (Box 12.1)
- The differential diagnosis of hemiplegic migraine includes transient ischemic attacks (TIAs), stroke, epilepsy with hemiparesis attributable to Todd's paresis, cerebrovascular disease (CADASIL, antiphospholipid antibody syndrome, vasculitis, HaNDL syndrome (headache associated with neurologic deficits and lymphocytic pleocytosis), central nervous system (CNS) infections (i.e., encephalitis, abscess), and mitochondrial diseases (MELAS)
- The main difference between hemiplegic migraine and typical aura with migraine headache is the presence of weakness/paralysis as an aura symptom. Hemiplegic migraine is the only migraine subtype in which weakness/paralysis occurs
- A diagnosis of hemiplegic migraine should be based on a thorough clinical history, general and neurologic exam and neuroimaging (MRI) to exclude secondary causes that may mimic hemiplegic migraine
- Genetic testing for FHM1, FHM2, and FMH2 is now commercially available

Box 12.1 Hemiplegic migraine – International Headache Society diagnostic criteria

1.2.4 Familial hemiplegic migraine (FHM)

Description:

Migraine with aura including motor weakness and at least one first- or second-degree relative has migraine aura including motor weakness

Diagnostic criteria:

A. At least 2 attacks fulfilling criteria B and C
B. Aura consisting of fully reversible motor weakness and at least one of the following:
   1. fully reversible visual symptoms including positive features (*eg*, flickering lights, spots or lines) and/or negative features (*ie*, loss of vision)
   2. fully reversible sensory symptoms including positive features (*ie*, pins and needles) and/or negative features (*ie*, numbness)
   3. fully reversible dysphasic speech disturbance
C. At least two of the following:
   1. at least one aura symptom develops gradually over ≥5 minutes and/or different aura symptoms occur in succession over ≥5 minutes
   2. each aura symptom lasts ≥5 minutes and <24 hours
   3. headache fulfilling criteria B–D for 1.1 *Migraine without aura* begins during the aura or follows onset of aura within 60 minutes
D. At least one first- or second-degree relative has had attacks fulfilling these criteria A–E
E. Not attributed to another disorder

1.2.5 Sporadic hemiplegic migraine (FHM)

Description:

Migraine with aura including motor weakness but no first- or second-degree relative has aura including motor weakness

Diagnostic criteria:

A. At least 2 attacks fulfilling criteria B and C
B. Aura consisting of fully reversible motor weakness and at least one of the following:
   1. fully reversible visual symptoms including positive features (*eg*, flickering lights, spots or lines) and/or negative features (*ie*, loss of vision)
   2. fully reversible sensory symptoms including positive features (*ie*, pins and needles) and/or negative features (*ie*, numbness)
   3. fully reversible dysphasic speech disturbance
C. At least two of the following:
   1. at least one aura symptom develops gradually over ≥5 minutes and/or different aura symptoms occur in succession over ≥5 minutes
   2. each aura symptom lasts ≥5 minutes and <24 hours
   3. headache fulfilling criteria B–D for 1.1 *Migraine without aura* begins during the aura or follows onset of aura within 60 minutes
D. No first- or second-degree relative has attacks fulfilling these criteria A–E
E. Not attributed to another disorder

■ Genetics

- Three different genetic mutations have been identified and have led to classification of familial hemiplegic migraine into three distinct subtypes: FHM1, FHM2, and FHM3

- Autosomal dominant inheritance with incomplete penetrance
- Poor genotype–phenotype relationship
- Sporadic mutations have been reported
- FHM1 – linkage to chromosome 19p13 (50% of cases)
  - Leads to a mutation in the *CACNA1A* gene, which codes for a P/Q type calcium channel
  - *CACNA1A* mutation also seen in episodic ataxia type 2, spinocerebellar ataxia type 6, and benign paroxysmal torticollis of infancy
- FHM2 – linkage to chromosome 1q23
  - Leads to a mutation in the *ATP1A2* gene which codes for a Na^+K^+ ATPase pump
  - *ATP1A2* mutations also seen in benign familial infantile convulsions and alternating hemiplegia of childhood
- FHM3 – linkage to chromosome 2q24
  - Leads to a mutation in the *SCN1A* gene, which codes for a voltage-gated sodium channel
  - *SCN1A* gene mutation also seen in generalized epilepsy with febrile seizures plus

■ Treatment

- There are no controlled trials of treatment in hemiplegic migraine
- Acute attacks should be treated at onset with aspirin or nonsteroidal antiinflammatory drugs (NSAIDs), oral or parental analgesics or opioids. Intranasal ketamine has been shown to abbreviate the aura and motor symptoms, but not prevent the headache. Parenteral magnesium sulfate, neuroleptics, and divalproex sodium have also been used in an attempt to alleviate the neurologic symptoms and terminate the headache

- Triptans and ergots are contraindicated because of their vasoconstrictive properties
- Case reports have suggested the utility of verapamil and acetazolamide in the prophylaxis of attacks. Topiramate and divalproex may also be used

■ Outcome

- Typically, attacks become less frequent and less severe after the age of 40
- In FHM1, progressive cerebellar symptoms may occur

■ Further reading

Black DR. Sporadic and familial hemiplegic migraine: diagnosis and treatment. *Seminar Neurol* 2006;**26**:208–216.

De Fusco M, Marconi R, Silvestri L, *et al.* Haploinsufficiency of ATP1A2 encoding the Na+/K+ pump alpha2 subunit associated with familial hemiplegic migraine type 2. *Nat Genet* 2003;**33**:192–196.

Dichigans M, Freilinger T, Eckstein G, *et al.* Mutation in the neuronal voltage-gated sodium channel SCN1A in familial hemiplegic migraine. *Lancet* 2005;**366**:371–377.

Ducros A, Dernier C, Joutel A, *et al.* The clinical spectrum of familial hemplegic migraine association with mutations in a neuronal calcium channel. *N Eng J Med* 2001;**345**:17–24.

Joutel A, Bousser MR, Biousse V, *et al.* A gene for familial hemiplegic migraine maps to chromosome 19. *Nat Genet* 1993;**5**:40–45.

Thomsen LL, Eriksen MK, Romer SF, *et al.* An epidemiological survey of hemiplegic migraine. *Cephalalgia* 2002;**22**:361–375.

Thomsen LL, Ostergaard E, Romer SF, *et al.* Sporadic hemiplegic migraine is an aetiologically heterogeneous disorder. *Cephalalgia* 2003;**23**:921–928.

13

Basilar-type migraine

■ Key points

- Basilar-type migraine consists of typical aura symptoms (visual, sensory, speech) plus additional atypical aura symptoms (bilateral visual disturbance, bilateral paresthesias, vertigo, ataxia, dysarthria, tinnitus, altered hearing, and decreased level of consciousness)
- Triptans and ergotamine are contraindicated in basilar-type migraine
- There is no proven effective prophylactic therapy for basilar-type migraine; however, calcium-channel blockers or anticonvulsants (such as topiramate or valproic acid) are frequently used

■ General overview

- Previously called basilar migraine, and renamed basilar-type migraine in the *International Classification of Headache Disorders 2nd edition* (ICHD-2). The name was changed to remove the implication that the basilar artery was responsible for the symptoms of basilar-type migraine
- Most common in children, teenagers and young adults
- The underlying pathophysiology of basilar-type migraine is unknown but may represent brainstem and/or bilateral hemispheric dysfunction, possibly due to spreading depression.

It is not considered, as previously thought, to be due to basilar artery spasm

- There is often a family history of migraine, migraine with aura, "atypical" migraine, "complicated" migraine, or basilar migraine

■ Clinical features

- Headache
  - Meets the criteria for the typical migraine with/without aura
  - Duration may be hours or days
  - Unilateral or bilateral; occipital location more common than in typical migraine with aura
  - Throbbing
  - Moderate to severe
- Associated features
  - Fully reversible typical aura symptoms including visual, sensory, and/or speech disturbances. The aura symptoms evolve gradually, often sequentially and typically last between 5 and 60 minutes
  - Motor symptoms/weakness are *not* a part of basilar-type migraine and if weakness is present, hemiplegic migraine or alternative diagnoses should be considered
  - In addition to typical aura symptoms, individuals with basilar-type migraine experience two or more of the following reversible aura symptoms lasting <60 minutes during an attack
    - Simultaneous bilateral visual symptoms in both the temporal and nasal fields of both eyes
    - Simultaneous bilateral paresthesias
    - Vertigo
    - Ataxia
    - Double vision
    - Dysarthria

- Decreased hearing
- Tinnitus
- Decreased level of consciousness
- Often associated with nausea and vomiting
- Patients may have photophobia and phonophobia
- Parietal lobe symptoms (disorders of body image and extrapersonal space, and disorientation) have been described
- Temporal lobe symptoms (depersonalizations, fear, automatisms) have been described

■ Diagnosis

- The diagnosis of basilar-type migraine is based on operational diagnostic criteria (Box 13.1)
- The differential diagnosis of basilar-type migraine includes hemiplegic migraine (see Chapter 12), typical migraine with aura (see Chapter 11), transient ischemic attack (TIA)/stroke, epilepsy, benign recurrent vertigo of childhood, vestibular migraine (migraine with associated vertigo), and epilepsy
- The main difference between hemiplegic migraine and basilar-type migraine is the presence of unilateral weakness/paralysis in hemiplegic migraine. Otherwise, there can be considerable overlap between these two migraine variants
- The main difference between the visual and sensory aura symptoms in basilar-type migraine and typical migraine with aura is that in basilar-type migraine the aura symptoms are bilateral. Also, in basilar-type migraine there are additional aura symptoms not commonly seen in typical migraine with aura
- The main difference between the symptoms of basilar-type migraine and those of a TIA or stroke is that in basilar-type migraine the aura symptoms are gradually progressive and additional symptoms often evolve sequentially. In patients with

Box 13.1 Basilar-type migraine – International Headache Society diagnostic criteria

Description:

Migraine with aura symptoms clearly originating from the brainstem and/or from both hemispheres simultaneously affected, but no motor weakness

Diagnostic criteria:

A. At least 2 attacks fulfilling criteria B–D

B. Aura consisting of at least two of the following fully reversible symptoms, but no motor weakness:
   1. dysarthria
   2. vertigo
   3. tinnitus
   4. hypacusia
   5. diplopia
   6. visual symptoms simultaneously in both temporal and nasal fields of both eyes
   7. ataxia
   8. decreased level of consciousness
   9. simultaneously bilateral paraesthesias

C. At least one of the following:
   1. at least one aura symptom develops gradually over ≥5 minutes and/or different aura symptoms occur in succession over ≥5 minutes
   2. each aura symptom lasts ≥5 and ≤60 minutes

D. Headache fulfilling criteria B–D for 1.1 *Migraine without aura* begins during the aura or follows aura within 60 minutes

E. Not attributed to another disorder

a TIA or stroke, the symptoms typically begin abruptly and with all symptoms occurring simultaneously rather than sequentially. Positive symptoms such as visual scintillations which are common in basilar-type migraine are uncommon in TIA and stroke

- Complicated attacks similar to basilar-type migraine have been described in patients with CADASIL (so-called CADASIL coma). Abnormal neuroimaging (high burden of T2/fluid attenuated inversion recovery [FLAIR] hyperintensity in the periventricular and deep white matter and particularly in the anterior temporal pole and external capsule) should raise suspicion for a secondary cause such as CADASIL
- Initially, neuroimaging (MRI with diffusion-weighted imaging sequences) is necessary to exclude an ischemic cause for the attacks. When occipitonuchal pain is prominent along with the symptoms, consideration should be given to vascular imaging to rule out a vertebral artery dissection

■ Treatment

- There is no approved treatment nor any well-studied treatment for basilar-type migraine
- Although a small case series has reported their safety, triptans and dihydroergotamine are contraindicated and should be avoided in basilar-type migraine due to the vasoconstrictive potential of these medications and the hypothetical risk of exacerbating the aura or precipitating infarction
- Acute attacks should be treated with NSAIDs, acetylsalicylic acid, and/or combination analgesics. Opioids, neuroleptic medications (e.g., prochlorperazine), magnesium sulfate, or parenteral divalproex sodium have also been used in the acute setting

- Prophylaxis with calcium-channel blockers has been advocated as first-line therapy; second-line therapy would be anticonvulsants such as topiramate or valproic acid. Acetazolamide has been used with some anecdotal success

■ Outcome

- Attacks of basilar-type migraine typically become less frequent and less severe later in adulthood and they invariably disappear, like hemiplegic migraine, before age 40. Often the attacks give way to typical migraine with or without aura

■ Further reading

Bickerstaff ER. Basilar artery migraine. *Lancet* 1961; **1**:15–17.

Caplan LP. Migraine and vertebrobasilar ischemia. *Neurology* 1991;**41**:55–61.

Klapper J, Mathew N, Nett R. Triptans in the treatment of basilar migraine and migraine with prolonged aura. *Headache* 2001;**42**:981–984.

La Spina I, Vignati A, Porazzi D. Basilar artery migraine: transcranial Doppler EEG and SPECT from the aura phase to the end. *Headache* 1997;**37**:43–47.

Panayiotopoulos CP. Basilar migraine? Seizures, and severe epileptic EEG abnormalities. *Neurology* 1980;**30**:1122–1125.

Sturzenegger MH, Meienberg O. Basilar artery migraine: a follow-up study of 82 cases. *Headache* 1985;**25**:408–415.

14

Episodic tension-type headache

■ Key points

- Tension-type headache is the most common type of headache worldwide
- Tension-type headaches rarely significantly interfere with function
- Individuals with episodic tension-type headache infrequently present to a medical practitioner with the chief complaint of headache
- Tension-type headache is one of the most common reasons for purchasing over-the-counter analgesics
- Little is known about the underlying pathogenesis of tension-type headache

■ General overview

- Tension-type headache is subdivided by the ICHD-2 into episodic tension-type headache (<1 per month), frequent tension-type headache (12–180 days per year), and chronic tension-type headache (≥180 days per year)
- One-year prevalence of tension-type headache ranges from 40% to over 80%

- Tension-type headache is slightly more common in females
- Prevalence peaks in the 30–39-year-old age group
- Tension-type headache does not cause workplace absenteeism but can cause presenteeism (decreased workplace effectiveness)

■ Clinical features

- Headache
  - Lasts from 30 minutes to 7 days
  - Bilateral
  - Pressing/tightening (non-pulsatile) quality
  - Mild to moderate in intensity
  - Not aggravated by routine physical activity such as walking or climbing stairs
- Associated features
  - Tension-type headaches are notable for their lack of associated features
  - May be associated with pericranial muscle tenderness
  - Nausea and vomiting do not occur in tension-type headache
  - Individuals with tension-type headache experience no more than one of photophobia or phonophobia and if present, hypersensitivity to external stimuli is not prominent

■ Diagnosis

- The diagnosis of tension-type headache is based on operational diagnostic criteria (Box 14.1)
- The differential diagnosis of episodic tension-type headache includes episodic migraine (see Chapter 11), cervicogenic headache (see Chapter 37), and secondary causes of headache
- The main difference between migraine and tension-type headache is that the tension-type headache is of lower severity

> ### Box 14.1 Episodic tension-type headache – International Headache Society diagnostic criteria
>
> *Diagnostic criteria:*
>
> A. At least 10 episodes occurring on <1 day per month on average (<12 days per year) and fulfilling criteria B–D
> B. Headache lasting from 30 minutes to 7 days
> C. Headache has at least two of the following characteristics:
>   1. bilateral location
>   2. pressing/tightening (non-pulsating) quality
>   3. mild or moderate intensity
>   4. not aggravated by routine physical activity such as walking or climbing stairs
> D. Both of the following:
>   1. no nausea or vomiting (anorexia may occur)
>   2. no more than one of photophobia or phonophobia
> E. Not attributed to another disorder

(mild to moderate), is more likely to be bilateral, lacks a throbbing component, is not affected by exertion, lacks prominent gastrointestinal symptoms (nausea, vomiting), and is associated with significantly less headache-related disability

- Tension-type headache is nondescript and featureless. It is notable that headaches secondary to space-occupying lesions such as brain tumors may present identical to tension-type headache. Correspondingly, all patients with new-onset chronic tension-type headache warrant neuroimaging
- Like cervicogenic headache, tension-type headache may be most prominent in the occipitonuchal region; however, cervicogenic headache is a strictly unilateral disorder

■ Treatment

- Treatment of tension-type headache includes lifestyle modifications to minimize headache occurrence, nonpharmacologic treatment modalities, and acute and prophylactic pharmacologic treatment

- An important early step in tension-type headache management is education about trigger factors and implementation of stress management and exercise to avoid/minimize tension-type headaches

- Acute tension-types headaches either resolve on their own or are managed with over-the-counter analgesics such as acetaminophen, NSAIDs, or acetylsalicylic acid. Combination products with caffeine are also effective

- Nonpharmacologic therapies include relaxation therapy, cognitive-behavioral therapy, and massage

- Prophylactic therapy is warranted when headaches are frequent, interfere with work, school or quality of life, and/or over-the-counter analgesic use is escalating (>10–15 days per month). Prophylactic options include tricyclic antidepressants such as amitriptyline and nortriptyline.

■ Outcome

- Most tension-type headaches occur sporadically (episodic or frequent tension-type headache)

- Up to 2%–3% of the population experience chronic tension-type headache

■ Further reading

Bigal ME, Lipton RB. Tension-type headache: classification and diagnosis. *Curr Pain Headache Rep* 2005;**9**:436–441.

Couch JR. The long-term prognosis of tension-type headache. *Curr Pain Headache Rep* 2005;**9**:423–429.

Jensen R, Bendtsen L. Tension-type headache: why does this condition have to fight for its recognition? *Curr Pain Headache Rep* 2006;**10**:454–458.

Lanaerts ME. Pharmacoprophylaxis of tension-type headache. *Curr Pain Headache Rep* 2005;**9**:442–447.

Lenaerts ME. Burden of tension-type headache. *Curr Pain Headache Rep* 2006;**10**:459–462.

15

Cluster headache

■ Key points

- Cluster headache is an excruciating, strictly unilateral, headache that usually last about 1 hour, and may recur up to 8 times per day
- Each attack is usually associated with cranial autonomic symptoms that are ipsilateral to the pain
- 20% of patients experience chronic cluster headache, diagnosed when headaches continue for 1 year without remission periods of 4 weeks or longer
- Chronic tobacco use and obstructive sleep apnea (OSA) are frequently comorbid
- MRI brain is required to exclude intracranial lesions, particularly those involving the pituitary and parasellar regions
- 100% oxygen, intranassal or parenteral triptans, corticosteroids, and verapamil are the treatments of choice

■ General overview

- Cluster headache is the prototype of the group of primary headache disorders referred to as trigeminal autonomic cephalalgias (TACs). The TACs are so-named because of the pain distribution (first division of trigeminal nerve) and accompanying ipsilateral cranial autonomic symptoms (lacrimation, conjunctival injection, rhinorrhea) (Table 15.1)

Table 15.1 The trigeminal autonomic cephalalgias

Feature	PH	SUNCT	Cluster
Sex (F:M)	2:1	1:2	1:3
Attack duration	~15 min	~1 min	60 min
Attack frequency (per day)	1–40	3–200	1–8
Treatment of choice	Indomethacin	Lamotrigine	Verapamil

PH, paroxysmal hemicrania; SUNCT, short-lasting unilateral neuralgiform headache attacks with conjunctival injection and tearing.

- Approximately 80% of patients with cluster headache experience attack (cluster) phases lasting 1–3 months, typically occurring once or twice per year, and remission phases, during which time attacks don't occur spontaneously and are not triggered
- 20% of patients develop chronic cluster headache, characterized by recurrent attacks for at least 1 year without remission periods of more than 4 weeks
- Patients experience 1–8 attacks per day, each lasting approximately 1 hour (15 minutes–3 hours). Nocturnal attacks are typical, but daytime attacks often occur, and the timing of attacks at or near the same time each day is characteristic
- Chronic tobacco use and OSA are frequent comorbidities
- Alcohol and high altitude are typical triggers.

■ Clinical features

- Headache
  - Strictly unilateral, often maximal around/behind the orbit
  - May begin or become referred to the temporal, lower facial, or occipital region
  - Extremely severe

- Often described as piercing, boring, or stabbing
  - Peaks within 3–5 minutes and lasts 60 minutes on average, with a range of 15–180 minutes
- Agitation
  - Restlessness and motor agitation is highly characteristic and seen in over 90% of patients. This is in contrast to migraine where activity aggravates the pain
- Autonomic symptoms
  - Autonomic features include lacrimation, rhinorrhea, conjunctival injection, ptosis, miosis, and facial or periorbital edema. Autonomic symptoms may occur bilaterally, but remain maximal on the side of the pain
- "Migrainous symptoms"
  - Symptoms classically linked with migraine occur in a significant number of patients with cluster headache and paroxysmal hemicrania (e.g., photophobia, phonophobia, nausea, aura)
  - Strictly ipsilateral photophobia and phonophobia occur in up to 50% of patients with TACs as opposed to <5% of patients with migraine
- Interparoxysmal pain and allodynia may occur in more than ⅓ of patients with any of the TACs, often in patients with a personal or family history of migraine
- Medication-overuse headache may be responsible for interparoxysmal headache in patients with TACs, particularly in those with a personal or family history of migraine

■ Diagnosis

- Clinical diagnosis is based on characteristic clinical features
- Cluster headache is distinguished from other TACs based on duration of individual attacks and frequency of attacks within a 24-hour period

- Physical exam
  - Persistent Horner syndrome may be seen in patients who have had recurrent attacks of cluster headache for years
- Imaging
  - MRI brain is indicated for patients with new-onset cluster headache, particularly if atypical clinical features are present or response to conventional therapy is absent
  - Special attention to the pituitary and parasellar region, as lesions in the areas may mimic cluster headache and other TACs
- Overnight polysomnography may be indicated if features of OSA are present. OSA is a frequent comorbid disorder

■ Treatment

Evidence-based guidelines for the treatment of cluster headache and other TACs are outlined in Tables 15.2 and 15.3. First-line treatments include the following:

- Acute treatment
  - 100% oxygen: 7–15 L per minute for 15 minutes using closed facemask
  - Triptans: sumatriptan 6 mg subcutaneous injection, sumatriptan 20 mg nasal spray, zolmitriptan 5 mg nasal spray
- Short-term prevention
  - Corticosteroids
    - 60 mg prednisone for 2–3 days, 50 mg for 2–3 days, with continued 10 mg dose decrements over each successive 2–3-day period (total 12–18-day treatment period)
    - Occipital nerve block (ipsilateral to pain)
      - 2.5 mL 0.5% bupivacaine plus 20 mg methylprednisolone

Table 15.2 Acute treatment for cluster headache and other trigeminal autonomic cephalalgias

Therapy	Treatment of choice		
	Cluster headache	Paroxysmal hemicrania	SUNCT syndrome
Acute	100% O_2, 7–15 L/min (A) Sumatriptan 6 mg subcutaneously (A) Sumatriptan 20 mg nasal (A) Zolmitriptan 5 mg nasal (A) Zolmitriptan 5 mg oral (B) Lidocaine intranasal (B) Octreotide (B)	None	None IV lidocaine (A)

A = effective; B = probably effective.

Table 15.3 Preventive treatment for cluster headache and other trigeminal autonomic cephalalgias

Therapy	Treatment of choice		
	Cluster headache	Paroxysmal hemicrania	SUNCT syndrome

Preventative	Verapamil (A)
	Steroids (A)
	  (PO/ONB)
	Lithium carbonate (B)
	Methysergide (B)
	Topiramate (B)
	Ergotamine
	  tartrate (B)
	Valproic acid (C)
	Melatonin (C)
	Gabapentin (C)
		Indomethacin (A)
		Verapamil (C)
		
		NSAIDs (C)
			Topiramate (B)
			Lamotrigine (C)
			
			Gabapentin (C)
			IV lidocaine (C)

A = effective; B = probably effective; C = possibly effective.

- Long-term prevention
  - Verapamil
    - Start with 80 mg three times daily; titrate to lowest effective dose up to 320 mg three times daily
    - Periodic ECG within 1–2 weeks after each dosage increase and bimonthly after highest dose established, to monitor for heart block
    - Patients should be counseled regarding the more common side-effects experienced with long-term use: gingival hyperplasia, constipation, and peripheral edema

■ Further reading

Bahra A, May A, Goadsby PJ. Cluster headache: a prospective clinical study in 230 patients with diagnostic implications. *Neurology* 2002;**58**:354–361.

Cohen AS, Matharu MS, Goadsby PJ. Trigeminal autonomic cephalalgias: current and future treatments. *Headache* 2007;**47**:969–980.

May A, Leone M, Afra J, *et al.* EFNS Task Force EFNS guidelines on the treatment of cluster headache and other trigeminal-autonomic cephalalgias. *Eur J Neurol* 2006;**13**:1066–1077.

16

Episodic paroxysmal hemicrania

■ Key points

- Similar to cluster headache with regards to attack characteristics and associated symptoms; however, attacks are shorter lasting and more frequent
- May be episodic (pain-free periods lasting >1month) or chronic (occurring daily or near-daily for >1 year); chronic paroxysmal hemicrania is more common than episodic paroxysmal hemicrania
- MRI brain with coronal gadolinium-enhanced sequences of the pituitary gland should be taken in all patients with suspected paroxysmal hemicrania
- Responds rapidly and completely to indomethacin (known as an indomethacin-responsive headache syndrome)

■ General overview

- A relatively rare primary headache syndrome recently included in the ICHD-2
- Slight female predominance
- Usual onset is early adulthood, mean age 36 years (range of 1–81 years reported)

■ Clinical features

- Headache
  - Typically exclusively unilateral (bilateral or alternating sides rarely reported)
  - Located maximally in the V1 region involving the orbital, supraorbital or temporal areas. However, pain may occur in any location (parietal, occipital)
  - Intensity is usually severe
  - Pain may be described as throbbing, pressure, stabbing, or boring
  - Attacks last for 2–30 minutes
  - Background pain occurs in up to 60% of patients
  - Frequency of >5 per day for more than half of the time (although periods with lower frequency may occur); average attack frequency 5–15 per day
  - Episodic with attacks lasting weeks or months; attacks lasting >1 year without remission or with remission periods lasting <1 month are referred to as chronic paroxysmal hemicrania. Chronic paroxysmal hemicrania is more common than episodic paroxysmal hemicrania (4:1)
- Associated features
  - Ipsilateral lacrimation and nasal congestion are most common
  - Other autonomic symptoms include rhinorrhea, conjunctival injection, eyelid edema, ptosis, miosis
  - Forehead or facial sweating occurs in more than 50% of patients
  - Ipsilateral sensation of ear-fullness or ear swelling occurs in ⅓
  - Photophobia and phonophobia occur in ⅔ of patients and may be unilateral. Nausea and vomiting occur in ⅓ and motion sensitivity in 50%
  - Bilateral autonomic symptoms have been reported rarely

- - Like cluster headache, agitation and restlessness occur in 80% of patients
- Triggers
  - Most attacks occur spontaneously
  - Attacks occur throughout the 24-hour period; there is no nocturnal predominance as in cluster headache

■ Diagnosis

- The diagnosis of paroxysmal hemicrania is based on operational diagnostic criteria (Box 16.1)

Box 16.1 Paroxysmal hemicrania – International Headache Society diagnostic criteria

Diagnostic criteria:

A. At least 20 attacks fulfilling criteria B–D

B. Attacks of severe unilateral orbital, supraorbital or temporal pain lasting 2–30 minutes

C. Headache is accompanied by at least one of the following:
  1. ipsilateral conjunctival injection and/or lacrimation
  2. ipsilateral nasal congestion and/or rhinorrhoea
  3. ipsilateral eyelid oedema
  4. ipsilateral forehead and facial sweating
  5. ipsilateral miosis and/or ptosis

D. Attacks have a frequency above 5 per day for more than half of the time, although periods with lower frequency may occur

E. Attacks are prevented completely by therapeutic doses of indomethacin

F. Not attributed to another disorder

3.2.1 *Episodic paroxysmal hemicrania*

Description:

Attacks of paroxysmal hemicrania occurring in periods lasting 7 days to 1 year separated by pain-free periods lasting ≥1 month

Diagnostic criteria:

A. Attacks fulfilling criteria A–F for 3.2 *Paroxysmal hemicrania*
B. At least two attack periods lasting 7–365 days and separated by pain-free remission periods of ≥1 month

3.2.2 *Chronic paroxysmal hemicrania (CPH)*

Description:

Attacks of paroxysmal hemicrania occurring for >1 year without remission or with remissions lasting <1 month

Diagnostic criteria:

A. Attacks fulfilling criteria A–F for 3.2 *Paroxysmal hemicrania*
B. Attacks recur over >1 year without remission periods or with remission periods lasting <1 month

- The differential diagnosis of paroxysmal hemicrania includes cluster headache (see Chapter 15), SUNCT syndrome (see Chapter 17), trigeminal neuralgia (see Chapter 19), and hemicrania continua (see Chapter 27)
- Clinically similar to episodic cluster headache; however, attacks have a higher frequency and shorter duration
- Clinically similar to SUNCT syndrome; however, paroxysmal hemicrania attacks have a longer duration and lower frequency, respond to indomethacin, and are not very susceptible to triggers

- When there is a dull interictal pain, paroxysmal hemicrania may resemble hemicrania continua; however, exacerbations with hemicrania continua are longer lasting with less robust autonomic features
- Secondary causes of paroxysmal hemicrania have been reported primarily with lesions in the pituitary region and posterior fossa
- Elimination of attacks with indomethacin is mandatory to make the diagnosis or paroxysmal hemicrania

■ Treatment

- Paroxysmal hemicrania responds completely to a trial of indomethacin. Response occurs within hours to days
- Usual starting dose is 25 mg three times daily with meals. Dose is doubled every 2 days if response is not complete until dose of 300 mg is reached. If response occurs, dose should be lowered by 25 mg every 3 days to determine the lowest effective dosage
- Given the propensity for gastrointestinal side-effects, mucosal protection is recommended
- Periodic attempts to lower the dose or discontinue indomethacin are recommended as remissions may occur
- When indomethacin is tolerated poorly, cyclo-oxygenase-2 inhibitors, acetylsalicylic acid, topiramate, or gabapentin may be used, though none have the consistent efficacy seen with indomethacin. Occipital nerve blockade may provide benefit

■ Outcome

- The natural history of paroxysmal hemicrania is not well known. In many individuals the attacks may last for years or decades requiring ongoing indomethacin prophylaxis; in some patients there is spontaneous remission

■ Further reading

Boes CJ, Swanson JW. Paroxysmal hemicrania, SUNCT and hemicrania continua. *Semin Neurol* 2006;**26**:260–270.

Cittadini E, Matharu MS, Goadsby PJ. Paroxysmal hemicrania: a prospective clinical study of thirty-one cases. *Brain* 2008;**131**:1142–1155.

Sjaastad O. Chronic paroxysmal hemicrania: from the index patient to the disease. *Curr Pain Headache Rep* 2006;**10**:295–301.

Sjaastad O, Dale I. Evidence for a new treatable headache entity. *Headache* 1974;**14**:105–108.

17

SUNCT syndrome

■ Key points

- SUNCT is the acronym for *s*hort-lasting, *u*nilateral, *n*euralgiform headache attacks with *c*onjunctival injection and *t*earing
- It is a subtype of the trigeminal autonomic cephalalgias (TACs)
- It is characterized by frequent (up to 200/day), strictly unilateral, severe, neuralgiform attacks in the ophthalmic division of the trigeminal nerve which are brief in duration (60 seconds) and occur in association with conjunctival injection and tearing
- Brain MRI with attention to the pituitary, parasellar region, and brainstem should be performed in all patients with suspected SUNCT syndrome
- Anticonvulsants (lamotrigine, gabapentin, topiramate, and carbamazepine) are effective in some patients. Parenteral lidocaine is effective, at least temporarily, in most patients with SUNCT

■ General overview

- A rare, primary headache syndrome recently included in the ICHD-2
- It shows slight male predominance
- The typical age of onset is 35–65 years (range 10–77 years)

■ Clinical features

- Headache
  - Typically unilateral (bilateral or alternating sides rarely reported)
  - Located maximally in the ophthalmic distribution (V1) of the trigeminal nerve (retro-orbital >forehead >temple) but can also radiate to the ipsilateral maxillary and mandibular divisions of the trigeminal nerve
  - Severe intensity in the majority and moderate in the minority
  - Pain is neuralgic (stabbing, shooting, lancinating, burning)
  - Attacks last for between 5 and 120 seconds. Most individuals are pain-free between attacks
  - Frequency of attacks can range from a few per day to several hundred per day
  - Typically no refractory period between attacks, unlike trigeminal neuralgia
- Associated features
  - Ipsilateral conjunctival injection and lacrimation most common
  - Other autonomic symptoms include rhinorrhea, nasal congestion, eyelid edema, ptosis, miosis, facial redness
  - "Migrainous" symptoms are not uncommon, particularly unilateral photophobia
  - In the appendix of the ICHD-2, a diagnostic entity entitled SUNA is proposed (short-lasting unilateral neuralgiform headache attacks with cranial autonomic symptoms) in order to remedy the fact that not all patients seem to experience conjunctival injection and tearing
- Triggers
  - Attacks may occur spontaneously or be triggered by tactile stimuli, similar to trigeminal neuralgia

■ Most common triggers are touching trigger zones (usually trigeminal-innervated territory) and mastication

■ Diagnosis

- The diagnosis of SUNCT syndrome is based on operational diagnostic criteria (Box 17.1)
- The differential diagnosis of SUNCT includes trigeminal neuralgia (see Chapter 19), primary stabbing headache (see Chapter 21), paroxysmal hemicrania, and cluster headache (see Chapter 15 and Fig. 17.1)
- Clinically similar to trigeminal neuralgia; however, SUNCT is almost always confined to V1 while trigeminal neuralgia is confined to V1 in less than 5% of patients. In addition, SUNCT attacks are longer, associated with autonomic symptoms, and have a refractory period
- Secondary causes of SUNCT have been reported with lesions occurring most commonly in the pituitary gland, parasellar region, and posterior fossa
- MRI brain with coronal enhanced images of the pituitary is required to rule out a secondary cause
- A trial of indomethacin is helpful to exclude an indomethacin-responsive headache

■ Treatment

- SUNCT is more refractory to treatment than other primary headache disorders
- The pharmacologic treatments with reported success in case reports and case series include: anticonvulsants (lamotrigine, gabapentin, carbamazepine, and topiramate), corticosteroids, and intravenous lidocaine

Box 17.1 SUNCT – International Headache Society diagnostic criteria

A. At least 20 attacks fulfilling criteria B–E
B. Attacks of unilateral, orbital, supraorbital or temporal stabbing or pulsating pain lasting 5–240 seconds
C. Pain is accompanied by ipsilateral conjunctival injection and lacrimation
D. Attacks occur with a frequency from 3 to 200 per day
E. Not attributed to another disorder

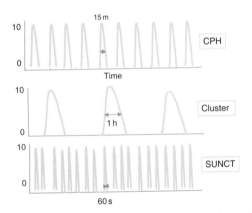

Fig. 17.1 Distinguishing the trigeminal autonomic cephalalgias by attack duration and frequency. CPH = chronic paroxysmal hemicrania

- Each of the pharmacologic treatments given here has been tried and reported to be generally or completely *ineffective*, although none of them has been adequately studied in a randomized, placebo-controlled study: simple analgesics, NSAIDs, cyclo-oxygenase-2 inhibitors, indomethacin, opiates, oxygen, triptans, ergots, calcium-channel blockers, benzodiazepines, tricyclic antidepressants, lithium, corticosteroids, and anticonvulsants (carbamazepine, phenytoin, valproic acid)

- Invasive surgical procedures involving the trigeminal nerve have had mixed success (percutaneous trigeminal ganglion rhizolysis and trigeminal root microvascular decompression) and should be considered only after all pharmacologic options have been exhausted. One case of medically intractable SUNCT responding to hypothalamic deep brain stimulation has been reported
- Local blockades (supraorbital, infraorbital, and greater occipital nerves) have been reported to be ineffective

■ Outcome

- The natural history of SUNCT is not well known. In many individuals the attacks seem to last years, decades, or may be lifelong

■ Further reading

Boes CJ, Swanson JW. Paroxysmal hemicrania, SUNCT and hemicrania continua. *Semin Neurol* 2006;**26**:260–270.

Cohen AS, Matharu MS, Goadsby PJ. Short-lasting unilateral neuralgiform headache attacks with conjunctival injection and tearing (SUNCT) or cranial autonomic features (SUNA) – a prospective clinical study of SUNCT and SUNA. *Brain* 2006;**129**:2746–2760.

Leroux E, Schwedt TH, Black DE, Dodick DW. Intractable SUNCT cured after resection of pituitary macroadenoma. *Can J Neurol Sci* 2006;**33**:411–413.

Matharu MS, Cohen AS, Boes CJ, Goadsby PJ. Short-lasting unilateral neuralgiform headache with conjunctival injection and tearing syndrome: a review. *Curr Pain Headache Rep.* 2003;**7**:308–318.

18

Chiari malformation headache

■ Key points

- Chiari malformation type I (CM-I) refers to at least 3–5 mm descent of the cerebellar tonsils below the foramen magnum (Fig. 18.1)
- Most patients are asymptomatic
- When present, headaches are often posterior and precipitated by coughing or Valsalva maneuver
- Cervical spinal cord syringomyelia, compression of the cervicomedullary junction, and obstructive hydrocephalus may be present
- MRI brain and cervical spinal cord are the imaging procedures of choice
- Treatment depends on the presence and severity of associated symptoms, but may include observation or surgical intervention

■ General overview

- CM-I consists of cerebellar tonsillar herniation through the foramen magnum of at least 3–5 mm
- It may be found in up to 5% of patients imaged for headache, and is most often an incidental finding and unrelated to the headache
- Patients with headaches that are precipitated by coughing or other Valsalva maneuvers (sneeze, bending, straining), especially those that are located in the posterior aspect of the

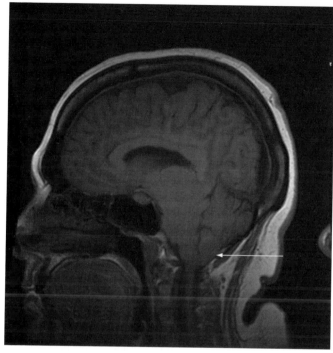

Fig. 18.1 Saggital MR view of Chiari malformation I: descent of the cerebellar tonsils through the foramen magnum.

head, should be evaluated for CM-I. Up to one half of patients with chronic recurrent headaches precipitated by cough may have CM-I

■ Clinical features

- Headache
  - Most common symptom (80%) in patients with symptomatic CM-I

- Most often occipital/suboccipital pain with possible radiation to the vertex, retroorbital region, or to the neck and shoulders
- Usually lasts minutes, but may last several hours
- Accentuated by cough, sneeze, Valsalva, and sudden changes in position
- Lower cranial nerve palsies
- Visual symptoms (sparks photopsias, diplopia, or transient visual blurring/loss of vision)
- Sensory disturbance
- Weakness

■ Diagnosis (Box 18.1)

- Physical exam
  - Scoliosis
  - Evidence of spinal cord syringomyelia
    - Loss of pain and temperature sensation in a "cape-like" distribution across the upper back, shoulders, and arms
- Imaging
  - MRI brain
    - Cerebellar tonsillar descent
    - Crowding of the subarachnoid space at the cervicomedullary junction
  - MRI cervical spinal cord
    - Syrinx
- Cerebrospinal fluid (CSF) flow studies if concern for cervicomedullary CSF obstruction

■ Treatment

- Asymptomatic, uncomplicated CM-I does not require specific treatment
- Indomethacin 25–300 mg

Box 18.1 Headache attributed to Chiari malformation type I – International Headache Society diagnostic criteria

A. Headache with ≥1 of the following and fulfilling criterion D:
  1. precipitated by cough and/or Valsalva manoeuvre
  2. protracted (hours to days) occipital and/or sub-occipital headache
  3. associated with symptoms and/or signs of brainstem, cerebellar and/or cervical cord dysfunction

B. Cerebellar tonsillar herniation as defined by one of the following on craniocervical MRI:
  1. ≥5 mm caudal descent of the cerebellar tonsils
  2. ≥3 mm caudal descent of the cerebellar tonsils plus evidence of crowding of the subarachnoid space in the area of the craniocervical junction

C. Evidence of posterior fossa dysfunction, based on ≥2 of the following:
  1. otoneurological symptoms and/or signs (eg, dizziness, disequilibrium, sensations of alteration in ear pressure, hypacusia or hyperacusia, vertigo, down-beat nystagmus, oscillopsia)
  2. transient visual symptoms (spark photopsias, visual blurring, diplopia or transient visual field deficits)
  3. demonstration of clinical signs relevant to cervical cord, brainstem or lower cranial nerves or of ataxia or dysmetria

D. Headache resolves within 3 months after successful treatment of the Chiari malformation

- Surgical decompression
  - Widely accepted indications:
    - Spinal cord syrinx
    - Cranial nerve deficits

- Gait instability
- Apnea
- Torticollis
- Surgical intervention in patients only with CM-I headache and no other symptoms is controversial and outcomes are difficult to predict

■ Further reading

Greenlee JDW, Donovan KA, Hasan DM, Menezes AH. Chiari I Malformation in the very young child: the spectrum of presentations and experience in 31 children under age 6 years. *Pediatrics* 2002;**110**:1212–1219.

Milhorat TH, Chou MW, Trinidad EM, *et al.* Chiari I malformation redefined: clinical and radiographic findings for 364 symptomatic patients. *Neurosurgery* 1999;**44**:1005–1017.

Stovner LJ. Headache associated with the Chiari Type I malformation. *Headache* 1993;**33**:175–181.

Weinberg JS, Freed DL, Sadock J, *et al.* Headache and Chiari I Malformation in the pediatric population. *Pediatr Neurosurg* 1998;**29**:14–18.

19

Trigeminal neuralgia

■ Key points

- Trigeminal neuralgia is a common neuralgic disorder, usually involving the 2nd and 3rd divisions (V2, V3) of the trigeminal nerve
- The pain is described as sharp, brief (usually 1–3 seconds), and lancinating. Typically, there are refractory periods between bouts of neuralgia
- Triggers include brushing the teeth, touching the face or gingiva, chewing, and talking
- The majority of cases are idiopathic; secondary causes include multiple sclerosis, intracranial tumor, and dental pathology
- Imaging modalities may be used to diagnose secondary trigeminal neuralgia and include MRI, and magnetic resonance angiography (MRA), and rarely conventional angiography
- Definitive evidence-based guidelines for the treatment of trigeminal neuralgia are not available for all therapies. Treatment options include observation, neuromodulation, analgesic medications, and surgical intervention

■ General overview

- Common neuralgic disorder in older individuals, usually after age 50, slight female preponderance

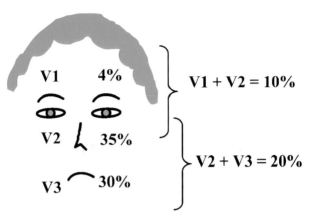

Fig. 19.1 Distribution of pain in trigeminal neuralgia.

- Severe unilateral pain, rarely bilateral; typically involves the V2 and V3 divisions of the trigeminal nerve (Fig. 19.1)
- Vascular cross-compression of fifth nerve outside the brainstem may be the most common "idiopathic" form, which is important in terms of therapy
- Any atypical clinical features, young age of onset or abnormal examination findings suggest the need for imaging, since up to 10% of patients have an intracranial lesion, such as a vascular lesion, tumor, or demyelinating disease

■ Clinical features (Box 19.1)

- Classical presentation
  - Jabbing unilateral facial pain usually in V2 or V3
  - Specific triggers with tactile input, such as brushing teeth
- Pain
  - Paroxysmal jabs of pain lasting only seconds
  - Pain of sudden onset, intense severity and superficial

Box 19.1 Clinical manifestations of trigeminal neuralgia

- Recurrent common neuralgic pain mainly in V2 and V3
- Jabbing and stabbing qualities
- Sudden intense pain but brief (seconds)
- Known trigger points in face and gums during brushing, chewing
- Pain-free between paroxysms
- Normal neurologic examination

- Pain-free intervals occurs between paroxysms, and can last seconds to hours
- Triggered by chewing, brushing teeth, talking, etc. and known trigger zones in nose, gums and face
- Onset
  - Mostly in people over 50 years of age
  - Infrequent in younger individuals – mostly in the setting of multiple sclerosis or other secondary causes
- Location
  - Second and third divisions of the trigeminal nerve
- Duration
  - Spontaneous remissions occur in 50% of patients
  - These can last up to 6 months or longer
- Associated pain
  - Some patients have background dull aching pain
  - Some have discomfort which precedes onset of true neuralgia; pre-trigeminal neuralgia is rare
- Other manifestations
  - No cranial nerve deficit is noted, and if a deficit is found, a secondary cause should be sought with appropriate neuroimaging

■ Diagnosis (Box 19.2)

- Physical exam
  - Neurologic exam
    - No abnormalities are detected usually. Some patients may complain of subjective facial sensory impairment
- Imaging
  - Imaging for trigeminal neuralgia may include: MRI to rule out mass, as well CTA or MRA to visualize any vascular loops or compression in the brainstem, and, rarely, conventional angiography
- MRA
  - The procedure of choice if available
  - Cross-compression of trigeminal sensory root should be looked for
- Conventional angiography
  - Gold standard for detection of vascular loop, but might be superseded by high-quality MRA or computed tomographic angiography (CTA)

Box 19.2 Classical trigeminal neuralgia – International Headache Society diagnostic criteria

A. Paroxysmal attacks of pain lasting from a fraction of a second to 2 minutes, affecting one or more divisions of the trigeminal nerve and fulfilling criteria B and C

B. Pain has at least one of the following characteristics:
   1. intense, sharp, superficial or stabbing
   2. precipitated from trigger areas or by trigger factors

C. Attacks are stereotyped in the individual patient

D. There is no clinically evident neurological deficit

E. Not attributed to another disorder

- MRI brain
  - Identify causes in brainstem or Meckel cave, or demyelination

■ Treatment

- Symptomatic
  - Anticonvulsant medications:
    - Carbamazepine is the standard medical treatment. Used in dosages similar to those used in epilepsy, starting low and building up slowly, with appropriate blood levels and blood tests to ensure no toxicity. Side-effects are usually tolerable but might limit use of higher dosages
    - Oxcarbazepine is likely similar in efficacy to carbamazepine and has fewer interactions and no need for blood levels
    - Gabapentin is a reasonable alternative with fewer serious side-effects but with a need for higher dosages; blood monitoring is not necessary
    - Topiramate is a third-line option
  - Other medications
    - Baclofen can be used alone or in combination with carbamazepine
  - Surgical intervention
    - Possible indications include:
      - Intractable trigeminal neuralgia
      - Known vascular lesion or secondary lesion
      - Intolerance of medications
    - Surgical options
      - Radiofrequency rhizotomy – sensory complications can occur

- Microvascular decompression of a vascular loop can be curative and has little risk in the modern era of neurosurgery
- Other surgical procedures are possible but used less frequently

■ Outcome

- Some patients have long spontaneous remissions
- Medication therapy is frequently sufficient
- Surgical options are curative in some cases

■ Further reading

Boecher-Schwarz HD, Bruehl K, Kessel G, *et al.* Sensitivity and specificity of MRA in the diagnosis of microvascular compression in patients with trigeminal neuralgia. A correlation of MRA and surgical findings. *Neuroradiology* 1998;**40**:88–95.

Eskandar EF, Barker G, 2nd, *et al.* Case records of the Massachusetts General Hospital. Case 21–2006. A 61-year-old man with left-sided facial pain. *N Eng J Med* 2006;**355**:183–188.

Hentschel K, Capobianco DJ, *et al.* Facial pain. *Neurologist* 2005;**11**:244–499.

Lance JW, Goadsby PJ. *Mechanisms and Management of Headache*. Elsevier, Philadelphia, 2005.

McLaughlin MR, Janetta PJ, Clyde BL, *et al.* Microvascular decompression of cranial nerves: Lessons learned after 4400 operations. *J Neurosurg* 1999;**90**:1–8.

Taha JM, Tew JM. Comparison of surgical treatments for trigeminal neuralgia: reevaluation of radiofrequency rhizotomy. *Neurosurgery* 1996;**38**: 865–871.

20

Subacute angle-closure glaucoma

■ Key points

- Patients with subacute angle-closure glaucoma may present primarily with headache
- Headaches of subacute angle-closure glaucoma may mimic migraine headache
- Early diagnosis and treatment is essential in order to reduce the risk of irreversible visual field loss
- Gonioscopy is necessary in the evaluation of this disorder

■ General overview

- There are two main types of primary glaucoma:
  - Wide-angle (open-angle)
  - Narrow-angle (angle-closure)
- Narrow-angle glaucoma
  - Apposition of the lens to the back of the iris, blocking movement of aqueous from the posterior to anterior chamber of the eye
  - Acute narrow-angle glaucoma
    - Presents emergently
      - Red eye
      - Painful eye – tender to touch
      - Impaired visual acuity

- Photophobia
- Visual halos
- Cornea – hazy
- Pupil – semi-dilated and fixed to light
- Nausea/vomiting
- Headache

- Subacute narrow-angle closure glaucoma
  - Presents less emergently with minimal to moderate intensity of symptoms
  - Patients with subacute narrow-angle closure glaucoma may present with episodic headache without ocular symptoms
  - More common in patients with hyperopia (far-sighted)

■ Clinical features

- Headache
  - Periodic attacks
    - Duration from several minutes up to 4 hours
    - More common in evening and nighttime during dim light
  - May mimic primary headache disorders such as migraine
    - Tends to be of shorter duration than migraine headaches
      - Several minutes up to 4 hours
    - Tends to occur later in life
      - Average – 6th to 7th decade
    - May be mild in intensity
    - Nonpulsating
    - No photophobia or phonophobia and not aggravated by routine activity
  - Location varies
    - Unilateral – most common
    - Frontal – most common
    - Temporal

- Hemifacial
- Diffuse
  - Pain may radiate to the eye
    - Primary ocular or periocular pain is not present in the majority
  - May be precipitated by emotional upset
  - Frequency of attacks varies
    - Most patients report daily headaches
    - May have intervals of several weeks between attacks
- Ophthalmologic symptoms
  - Ocular discomfort
  - Visual symptoms
    - Only present in about ⅓ of patients
    - Blurred vision
    - Colored halos around lights
- Nausea/vomiting

■ Diagnosis

- Diagnosis depends on ophthalmologic evaluation to include gonioscopy
  - Gonioscopy – placing a mirrored prism on the surface of the eye in order to visualize the anatomy of the peripheral cornea, trabecular meshwork, and iris root
  - Gonioscopy is not part of the routine ophthalmologic examination and thus must be specifically requested
- Eye exam
  - Eye white
  - Anterior chamber shallow
  - Cornea clear
    - Epithelial edema if tension present
  - Pupil normal
    - May be slightly dilated and sluggish to react if tension is elevated

- Optic disk normal
  - Cupping and atrophy in late stages of the disease
- Tension
  - Normal between attacks
  - Elevated during attacks
    - Generally less than 50mm
- Gonioscopy
  - Convexity of the iris
  - Narrow angle
  - If done when tension is elevated, angle closure is visualized
- Perimetry
  - Normal
  - Glaucomatous field defects
    - Arcuate scotoma

Treatment

- Pilocarpine hydrochloride drops
  - Alleviation of symptoms
    - Provides evidence that headache and other symptoms are secondary to subacute angle-closure glaucoma
- Laser iridotomy
  - Definitive treatment
  - Creates an opening in the iris allowing for aqueous flow from the posterior to anterior chamber

Outcome

- In the majority of patients, the symptoms resolve following laser iridotomy
- If diagnosis is delayed, permanent visual field deficits may occur

■ Further reading

Chandler PA, Trotter RR. Angle-closure glaucoma: subacute types. *Trans Am Ophthalmol Soc* 1954;**52**:265–290.

Khaw PT, Shah P, Elkington AR. Glaucoma 1: diagnosis. *Br Med J* 2004;**328**:97–99.

Lewis J, Fourman S. Subacute angle-closure glaucoma as a cause of headache in the presence of white eye. *Headache* 1998;**38**:684–686.

Nesher R, Epstein E, Stern Y, *et al.* Headaches as the main presenting symptom of subacute angle closure glaucoma. *Headache* 2005;**45**:172–176.

Shindler KS, Sankar PS, Volpe NJ, Piltz-Seymour JR. Intermittent headaches as the presenting sign of subacute angle-closure glaucoma. *Neurology* 2005;**65**:757–758.

21

Primary stabbing headache

■ Key points

- Primary stabbing headache (PSH) is characterized by spontaneous, unpredictable, paroxysmal attacks of fleeting head pain that is stabbing in quality
- The majority of attacks last less than 1 second and while any location of the head can be involved, the ophthalmic distribution of the trigeminal nerve is most common
- Frequently associated with other primary headache disorders, but may be the presentation of secondary disorders
- For attacks occurring frequently the treatment of choice is indomethacin

■ General overview

- PSH was previously known as ophthalmodynia periodica, ice pick headache, jabs and jolts syndrome, and idiopathic stabbing headache
- Lifetime prevalence of PSH is less than 2%
- Frequently associated with other primary headache disorders including migraine (40%), tension-type headache, and the trigeminal autonomic cephalalgias

- Secondary causes of stabbing headache include structural intracranial lesions (meningiomas, pituitary tumors), giant cell arteritis, cranial and ocular trauma, herpes zoster, and intraocular pressure elevation

■ Clinical features

- Ultra-short paroxysms of stabbing pain (1–10 seconds)
- Age at onset is 12–70 (mean 47 years). Female predominance ranges from 1.5:1 to 6.6:1
- Usually unilateral, in the ophthalmic distribution of the trigeminal nerve
- Sites less commonly affected by the pain include the facial, temporal, parietal, retroauricular, and occipital regions of the head
- The frequency of attacks is quite variable, ranging from 1 attack per year to 50 attacks daily
- Frequent attacks (>80% of days) occur in less than 14% of patients
- Mostly, attacks occur throughout the day and evening with irregular intervals between the attacks

■ Diagnosis (Box 21.1)

- Differential diagnosis includes:
  - SUNCT – individual attacks are longer (10–300 seconds), associated with conjunctival injection and tearing, and are exclusively unilateral and confined to the orbitotemporal region.
  - Trigeminal neuralgia – uncommon to be confined to V1 distribution (4%), whereas involvement of V2/V3 is rare in PSH. Triggers associated with trigeminal neuralgia, whereas PSH is spontaneous and not associated with triggers
  - Secondary causes (see above)

> **Box 21.1** Primary stabbing headache – International
> Headache Society diagnostic criteria
>
> *Description:*
>
> Transient and localized stabs of pain in the head that occur
> spontaneously in the absence of organic disease of underlying
> structures of the cranial nerves
>
> *Diagnostic criteria:*
>
> A. Head pain occurring as a single stab or a series of stabs and
>   fulfilling criteria B and C
> B. Exclusively or predominantly felt in the distribution of the first
>   division of the trigeminal nerve
> C. Stabs last for up to a few seconds and recur with irregular
>   frequency ranging from one to many per day
> D. No accompanying symptoms
> E. Not attributed to another disorder

■ Investigations

- Usually not necessary, unless there is suspicion for a
  secondary cause based on history and examination, or
  the attacks are frequent, strictly unilateral or confined to
  a focal site on the head, or the patient does not respond
  to indomethacin

■ Treatment

- Acute treatment of PSH is not practical because of the ultra-
  short duration of attacks. Prophylactic therapy is rarely
  required

- Indomethacin (25–75 mg three times daily) provides complete or partial relief in most but not all patients with frequent and daily attacks
- Melatonin (3–12 mg/day) and gabapentin (400 mg twice daily) may also be effective

■ Further reading

Dodick DW. Indomethacin responsive headache syndromes. *Curr Pain Head Rep* 2004;**8**:19–28.

Pareja JA, Rujiz J, Deisla C, *et al*. Idiopathic stabbing headache (jabs and jolt syndrome). *Cephalalgia* 1996;**16**:93–96.

Rozen TD. Melatonin as treatment for idiopathic stabbing headache. *Neurology* 2003;**61**:865–866.

22

Primary headache associated with sexual activity

■ Key points

- Primary headache associated with sexual activity can occur with sexual intercourse or masturbation
- Most commonly, severe headaches of sudden onset (thunderclap headaches) occur at the time of orgasm
- The differential diagnosis includes the usual causes of thunderclap headache including subarachnoid hemorrhage, arterial dissection, stroke, and cerebral vasoconstriction
- Clinical course ranges from a single event to recurrent events over weeks or years
- Treatment is preventive for those with frequent or recurrent attacks and includes indomethacin, β-blockers, and calcium-channel blockers
- Vasoconstrictive drugs, such as triptans and ergotamine, should be avoided

■ General overview

- Primary headache associated with sexual activity was previously known as benign sex headache, coital headache, benign vascular sexual headache, and benign orgasmic headaches
- It may occur during masturbation as well as sexual intercourse.
- The lifetime prevalence is 1%. In subspecialty clinics, 0.2%–1.3% of all patients report these headaches

■ Clinical features

- Two types
  - Pre-orgasmic (20%): resemble tension-type headache; bilateral, generalized dull ache involving the head and neck and/or tightness of the muscles of the jaw and neck occurring during sexual activity. Begin as sexual excitement builds, and can be prevented or reduced by deliberate muscle relaxation
  - Orgasmic (80%): the headaches begin abruptly, at the moment of orgasm, and may be caused by or associated with an increase in blood pressure. The pain is explosive, severe, occipital, or generalized, and may be associated with nausea and vomiting. These headaches typically last from 1 minute to 3 hours
- Clinical course may be unpredictable. Headaches associated with sexual activity may recur over a short period of time (weeks), occur infrequently over years, or occur once never to recur again
- If the headaches occur repeatedly over the course of 1–2 weeks, noninvasive cerebral angiography should be performed to exclude the possibility of reversible cerebral vasoconstriction syndrome

■ Diagnosis

- Differential diagnosis includes all potential causes of thunderclap headache including:
  - Subarachnoid hemorrhage
  - Cerebral venous sinus thrombosis
  - Ischemic or hemorrhagic stroke
  - Reversible cerebral vasoconstriction
  - Arterial dissection

- CSF leak
- Hypertensive encephalopathy with or without posterior reversible encephalopathy syndrome (PRES)
- Investigations are required in patients presenting for the first time with acute headache associated with sexual activity
  - CT without contrast
  - If CT is negative, lumbar puncture for CSF analysis and opening pressure
  - If CT and CSF are normal, MRI brain with gadolinium and angiography (MRA or CTA) of the head and neck

■ Treatment

- Acute treatment is often not necessary because of the self-limited, short-lasting nature of the headache. Vasoactive drugs such as triptans and ergotamine derivatives should be avoided because of the association with arterial hypertension and the potential for secondary causes such as arterial dissection or cerebral vasoconstriction
- Preemptive treatment with indomethacin 50–100 mg taken 30–60 minutes prior to sexual activity may prevent attacks in individuals experiencing frequent or recurrent attacks
- Prophylaxis for people with recurrent attacks may include indomethacin 25–50 mg three times daily with meals, β-blockers such as propranolol 40–240 mg daily, metoprolol 25–50 mg, or atenolol 25–50 mg per day. Caution as β-blockers may be associated with impotence in males
- Calcium-channel blockers may also be useful: diltiazem 40–60 mg three times daily or verapamil 60–80 mg three times daily

■ Further reading

Evans RW, Pascual J. Orgasmic headaches: clinical features, diagnosis and management. *Headache* 2000;**40**:491–494.

Frese A, Eikermann A, Frese K, *et al*. Headache associated with sexual activity. Demography, clinical features, and comorbidity. *Neurology* 2003; **61**:796–800.

23

Primary cough headache

■ Key points

- Primary cough headache (PCH) is characterized by a sudden, severe, diffuse headache that is short lasting (<30 minutes) and is provoked by cough or other Valsalva maneuvers
- The disorder is most common in middle-aged and elderly men
- Approximately 50% of patients presenting with cough headache have a secondary cause
- MRI brain is necessary in all patients to exclude secondary causes
- Treatment of choice in PCH is indomethacin

■ General overview

- The lifetime prevalence of PCH is 1%
- It usually affects men over the age of 40; mean age of onset is 67 years
- Mechanism is not clear but hypotheses include: increased intracranial venous pressure, hypersensitive pressure receptors in the cerebral venous system, and reduced volume of the posterior cranial fossa

■ Clinical features

- Headache
  - Often sudden, severe, diffuse

- Precipitated by coughing or other Valsalva maneuvers such as sneezing, straining, laughing, and bending
  - Duration is typically 1 second to 30 minutes. A dull headache may persist for several hours
- Associated symptoms such as nausea, emesis, photophobia, and visual symptoms are generally absent

Differential diagnosis

- Space-occupying lesion
- Chiari malformation
- Sinusitis
- Structural mass that obstructs CSF flow (e.g., colloid cyst of the third ventricle)
- CSF leak
- Secondary causes should be suspected when:
  - Young age (<50 years)
  - Female
  - Headache lasts longer than 30 minutes
  - Neurologic symptoms or signs are present

Investigations

- MRI brain with gadolinium in all patients because of the high frequency of secondary causes
- If CSF leak is suspected clinically or based on radiographic findings, the appropriate investigations to exclude this disorder are indicated

Treatment

- Indomethacin 25–75 mg three times daily with meals or sustained-release indomethacin 75 mg is the treatment of choice in patients with persistent symptoms

- There are anecdotal case reports of patients responding to naproxen sodium, acetazolamide, methysergide, dihydroergotamine, propranolol, and topiramate
- Lumbar puncture with removal of ~40 mL of cerebrospinal fluid may be effective

■ Further reading

Pascual J. Primary cough headache. *Curr Pain Head Rep* 2005;**9**:272–276.

Pascual J, Iglesias F, Oterino A, *et al.* Cough, exertional and sexual headaches: an analysis of 72 benign and symptomatic cases. *Neurology* 1996;**46**:1520–1524.

Raskin NH. The cough headache syndrome: treatment. *Neurology* 1995;**45**:1784.

SECTION 3
Chronic daily headaches

24

Introduction to the chronic daily headaches

Chronic daily headache (CDH) is a symptom rather than a diagnosis. CDH refers to the presence of headache on ≥15 days per month for ≥3 months. Worldwide, 3%–5% of the general population has CDH. CDH occurs in children, teenagers, adults, and the elderly. Patients with CDH have significantly diminished health-related quality of life and decreased physical, social, and occupational functioning and mental health.

Fortunately, in the vast majority of individuals, CDH is attributable to a benign primary headache disorder; nonetheless, clinicians need to be vigilant for secondary causes of chronic headaches in their patients. The differential diagnosis of CDH is lengthy as there are literally hundreds of different causes. An overview of the common primary and secondary causes of CDH is presented in Box 24.1. The following chapters in this section review 15 of the most common and/or important causes of CDH.

A thorough history is the most critical aspect of the evaluation and leads to the diagnosis in the vast majority of cases. Occasionally, findings on examination unexpectedly suggest a secondary cause for the CDH. There are several "red flags" that increase the likelihood that the CDH is secondary to an underlying cause. These "red flags" are presented in Box 24.2.

Box 24.1 Causes of chronic daily headache

Primary causes

- Chronic migraine[1]
- Chronic tension-type headache[1]
- New daily persistent headache
- Chronic cluster
- Hemicrania continua

Secondary causes

Medication-related:

- Medication-overuse headache[1]
- Drug side-effects

Post-traumatic:

- Headache attributable to head injury
- Headache attributable to neck injury or whiplash

Disorders of intracranial pressure:

- Increased intracranial pressure (primary or secondary tumor, idiopathic intracranial hypertension, hydrocephalus)
- Decreased intracranial pressure (spontaneous intracranial hypotension, postlumbar puncture headache)

Structural:

- Headache attributable to cervical spine disorders
- Headache attributable to temporomandibular joint (TMJ)/dental pathology

Cranial neuralgias:

- Trigeminal neuralgia
- Occipital neuralgia

Vascular:

- Subdural hematoma
- Giant cell arteritis
- Ischemic or hemorrhagic stroke
- Venous sinus thrombosis
- Arterial dissection
- Severe arterial hypertension

Infectious:

- Meningitis (tuberculosis, fungal, parasitic)
- Sinusitis (sphenoid sinusitis)

Metabolic:

- Obstructive sleep apnea, hypoxia, hypercarbia, carbon monoxide
- Thyroid disease

[1]Represents the most common primary and secondary causes of chronic daily headache.

Box 24.2 Chronic daily headache – "red flags" on history or physical examination

Red flags on history

Onset age >50 years

- Consider temporal arteritis, brain tumor (primary or secondary), or subdural hematoma

Precipitated or exacerbated by positional changes, Valsalva, bending, or coughing

- If worse when standing – think spontaneous intracranial hypotension
- If worse when supine or with Valsalva – think increased intracranial pressure and/or posterior fossa abnormality

History of cancer, immunocompromise, or human immunodeficiency virus (HIV)

- Be wary of metastatic disease or intracranial infection

Progressive headache or escalating medication requirements

- Re-evaluate original diagnosis, and consider a secondary cause
- Be wary of caffeine and/or medication overuse

Red flags on examination

Focal neurologic symptoms or findings

- Any accompanying neurologic symptom or neurologic sign suggests a secondary cause and warrants investigation (i.e., change in mentation or personality, optic disk swelling, field cut, focal weakness, incoordination, etc.)

Presence of systemic signs or symptoms

- Chronic meningitis (tuberculosis, fungal, or parasitic infection)
- Sinusitis (note sphenoid sinusitis may occur without nasal symptoms)
- Vasculitis (primary central nervous system [CNS] or secondary to other inflammatory/rheumatologic conditions)
- Temporal arteritis (fatigue, polymyalgia rheumatica, jaw claudication, scalp tenderness)

All patients with CDH of less than 6 months duration require an unenhanced computed tomography (CT) scan of the brain. If there are any "red flags" on history, any abnormalities on physical exam, or if the headache is not easily classifiable as a primary headache syndrome, further workup is required (i.e., blood tests, CT with contrast or magnetic resonance imaging [MRI]) with gadolinium, neurologic and/or ophthalmologic consultation).

It is important to remember that many secondary causes of CDH can be missed by stopping the investigation after a "normal" CT head (i.e., temporal arteritis, intracranial hypertension, intracranial hypotension, chronic subdural hematoma, etc).

25

Chronic migraine headache

■ Key points

- Chronic migraineurs have headaches on ≥15 days/month with migraine headaches on ≥8 of these days
- Chronic migraine affects 2%–3% of the general population
- Each year, between 3% and 14% of patients with episodic migraine transform to chronic migraine
- Chronic migraine must be differentiated from other forms of chronic daily headache (CDH) including chronic tension-type headache (CTTH), cluster headache, medication-overuse headache (MOH), hemicrania continua, and new daily persistent headache (NPDH)
- The treatment of chronic migraine consists of a multimodal approach, combining pharmacologic and nonpharmacologic prophylactic and abortive therapies

■ General overview

- The chronic migraineur has headaches (tension-type and/ or migraine) on ≥15 days per month for >3 months. On ≥8 days per month the headache meets standard criteria for the pain and associated symptoms of migraine or the headache responds to a triptan or ergot abortive medication (see Box 25.1)

Box 25.1 Chronic migraine – International Headache Society diagnostic criteria

A. Headache (tension-type and/or migraine) on ≥15 days/month for ≥3 months

B. Occurring in a patient who has had at least 5 attacks fulfilling criteria for migraine without aura

C. On ≥8 days per month for ≥3 months headache has fulfilled criteria C1 and/or C2 below

  1. Has ≥2 of a–d
     a. unilateral location
     b. pulsating quality
     c. moderate or severe pain
     d. aggravation by or causing avoidance of routine physical activity and ≥1 of a or b
     a. nausea and/or vomiting
     b. photophobia and phonophobia
  2. Treated and relieved by triptan(s) or ergot before the expected development of C1 above

D. No medication overuse and not attributed to another causative disorder

- 4% of the general population has headaches on ≥15 days/month (CDHs), about ½ of whom have chronic migraine
- Chronic migraine results in substantial disability, decreased quality of life, and impaired physical, social, and occupational functioning
- The World Health Organization considers chronic migraine among the most disabling illnesses, causing disability on a par with that secondary to quadriplegia, dementia, and active psychosis

■ Clinical features

- Many patients with chronic migraine have daily or near-daily mild to moderate headaches with superimposed episodic headaches of greater severity
- Environmental sensitivities (e.g., photophobia, phonophobia, motion sensitivity) may be present to a mild degree between headaches and during milder headaches, with a tendency to increase in intensity during full-blown severe migraine headaches
- Chronic migraine is frequently associated with several other disorders including:
  - Depression
  - Anxiety
  - Fatigue
  - Myofascial pain
  - Sleep disorders/snoring
  - Gastrointestinal disorders

■ Transformation from episodic migraine

- In the general population, 3% of episodic migraineurs transform to chronic migraine each year
- In a clinic-based population, 14% of episodic migraine patients transform to chronic migraine each year
- In addition, 6% of people with infrequent episodic migraine (2–104 headache days/year) transform to frequent episodic migraine (105–179 headache days/year) each year
- Non-modifiable risk factors for transformation to chronic migraine include:
  - Female sex
  - Low socioeconomic status

- Younger age
- History of head/neck injury
- Potentially modifiable risk factors for transformation to chronic migraine include:
  - Obesity
  - Overuse of abortive migraine medications
  - Stress
  - Sleep disorders/snoring
  - Depression
  - High caffeine intake

■ Diagnosis

- The diagnosis of chronic migraine is based on headache characteristics. No specific diagnostic tests are required to make the diagnosis
- The diagnostic criteria for chronic migraine are shown in Box 25.1
- Like the evaluation of all headaches, the healthcare provider must take a careful medical and headache history and perform necessary physical and neurologic exams in search of features that increase the suspicion for a secondary headache disorder. If any of these characteristics are present, diagnostic tests may be necessary to differentiate chronic migraine from a secondary headache disorder. (See Chapter 24 for a description of headache "red flags" which increase the suspicion for a secondary headache disorder)
- Headache types most commonly considered in the differential diagnosis of chronic migraine include: chronic tension-type headache (see Chapter 26), hemicrania continua (see Chapter 27), episodic/chronic cluster headache (see Chapter 15), medication-overuse headache (see Chapter 35), and new daily persistent headache (see Chapter 28)

- Chronic tension-type headache: Although chronic migraineurs are likely to have some tension-type headaches, they must also have ≥8 days/month with headaches meeting diagnostic criteria for migraine
- Hemicrania continua: Chronic migraine may be easily differentiated from hemicrania continua when pain is bilateral and episodic. However, some patients with chronic migraine have continuous one-sided pain. Typically, hemicrania continua is associated with ipsilateral autonomic features (reddening of the eye, tearing from the eye, nasal congestion, or rhinorrhea) that occur during severe episodic exacerbations of pain. Autonomic features are absent or less prominent in the typical migraine patient. However, when there is diagnostic uncertainty in a patient with primary continuous one-sided headaches, an indomethacin trial may be required to differentiate hemicrania continua from chronic migraine. The patient with hemicrania continua has complete response to sufficient doses of indomethacin
- Cluster headache: Cluster headaches can be differentiated from migraine due to their exclusive unilateral location, presence of substantial ipsilateral autonomic features, shorter duration of individual headaches, male predominance, and tendency to cause increased activity/agitation during the headache. Typically, the chronic cluster headache patient is pain-free between individual headache attacks, each lasting 15–180 minutes
- Medication overuse headache: Patients with headaches on ≥15 days/month frequently overuse abortive medications. Recognition of medication overuse is essential in the patient with frequent headaches since successful treatment often depends on reduction in medication use

- New daily persistent headache: NDPH refers to a daily headache that has been unremitting from onset, or unremitting within <3 days of onset, and has been present for >3 months. Differentiating it from chronic migraine, pain is often bilateral, nonthrobbing, mild or moderate in severity, and not aggravated by routine activities. There is absence of or only mild photophobia, phonophobia, or nausea. There is high suspicion for a secondary headache disorder in the patient with new daily persistent headache

- Patients should be screened for symptoms suggestive of disorders that are frequently comorbid with chronic migraine (as listed above)

■ Treatment

- Lifestyle modification
  - Limit caffeine intake
  - Regular meals
  - Regular sleep schedule
  - Avoidance of other migraine triggers as possible:
    - Stress
    - Alcohol
    - Cigarette smoke
    - Dietary triggers
- Prophylactic therapy
  - Although fewer medications have been systematically investigated for their use in prevention of chronic migraine than for episodic migraine, the prophylactic therapy for both migraine types is similar. The most widely used medications for migraine prophylaxis are:
    - Antihypertensives
      - β-Blockers

- Calcium-channel blockers
- Antidepressants
  - Tricyclics
  - Fluoxetine
- Anticonvulsants
  - Topiramate
  - Valproic acid
  - Gabapentin
- Vitamins/supplements
  - Riboflavin
  - Magnesium
  - Feverfew
  - Butterbur
- Botulinum toxin
- Other pharmacologic treatments that could be considered (but have less evidence supporting their use) include:
  - Pregabalin
  - Zonisamide
  - Levetiracetam
  - Memantine
  - Coenzyme Q-10
  - Angiotensin-converting enzyme inhibitors
  - Angiotensin receptor blockers
  - Other selective serotonin reuptake inhibitors
  - Serotonin-norepinephrine reuptake inhibitors
- Abortive migraine therapy
  - Not different from abortive therapy for episodic migraine (see Chapter 11)
    - Nonsteroidal anti-inflammatory drugs (NSAIDs)
    - Triptans
    - Ergotamines
    - Butalbital-containing analgesics

- Antiemetics
  - Limit use of abortive medications to an average of ≤3 days/week
    - Generally means not treating mild to moderate non-migraine headaches with abortive medications
- Physical therapy
  - Indicated if there is evidence for a myofascial component to the patient's pain or evidence for myofascial headache triggers
- Biobehavioral therapy
  - Biofeedback, relaxation therapy, and cognitive-behavioral therapy may be useful adjunctive therapies
- Breaking the headache cycle
  - Patients with daily headaches or status migraine may require acute interventions to break the headache cycle
  - Outpatient and inpatient protocols may be used
  - Examples of frequently used medications are:
    - Intravenous or injectable dihydroergotamine (DHE)
    - Intravenous or oral corticosteroids
    - Injectable, intravenous or oral NSAIDs
    - Intravenous magnesium
    - Intravenous neuroleptics
    - Intravenous valproic acid

■ Outcome

- Patients with chronic migraine can revert to an episodic migraine pattern
- Factors associated with reversion to episodic migraine include good compliance with prophylactic medications, avoidance of abortive medication overuse, and regular exercise
- In a clinic-based sample of patients being treated for chronic migraine, 70% reverted to episodic migraine within 1 year

- In a population-based sample, just over 50% of patients reverted within 1 year

■ Further reading

Bigal ME, Lipton RB. Modifiable risk factors for migraine progression. *Headache* 2006;**46**:1334–1343.

Harwood RH, Sayer AA, Hirschfeld M. Current and future worldwide prevalence of dependency, its relationship to total population, and dependency ratios. *Bull World Health Organ* 2004;**82**:251–258.

Mathew NT. The prophylactic treatment of chronic daily headache. *Headache* 2006;**46**:1552–1564.

Scher AI, Stewart WF, Liberman J, Lipton RB. Prevalence of frequent headache in a population sample. *Headache* 1998;**38**:497–506

Scher AI, Stewart WF, Ricci JA, Lipton RB. Factors associated with the onset and remission of chronic daily headache in a population-based study. *Pain* 2003;**106**:81–89.

Seok JI, Cho HI, Chin-Sang C. From transformed migraine to episodic migraine: reversion factors. *Headache* 2006;**46**:1186–1190.

26

Chronic tension-type headache

■ Key points

- In the general population, chronic tension-type headache (CTTH) is the most common cause of chronic daily headache (CDH)
- Little is known about the underlying pathogenesis of tension-type headache
- Avoidance of trigger factors, nonpharmacologic treatment interventions, and/or pharmacologic prophylaxis can help a significant proportion of individuals with CTTH

■ General overview

- Tension-type headache is consider by the *International Classification of Headache Disorders 2nd edition* (ICHD-2) to be chronic (i.e., CTTH) when it occurs on ≥15 days per month on average for >3 months (≥180 days per year)
- 1-year prevalence of CTTH ranges from 2% to 4%
- Depression is observed with higher prevalence in patients with CTTH
- Tension-type headache is a common and important cause of workplace presenteeism (decreased workplace effectiveness/efficiency)

■ Clinical features

- Headache
  - ■ May last for hours or be continuous
  - ■ Usually bilateral; may be holocranial, frontotemporal and/or occipitonuchal
  - ■ Pressing, tightening, dull ache, "tight band," "cap," and "weight" are common descriptions of the quality of the pain
  - ■ Mild to moderate in intensity
  - ■ Not aggravated by routine physical activity such as walking or climbing stairs
- Associated features
  - ■ Tension-type headaches are notable for their lack of associated features
  - ■ May be associated with pericranial muscle tenderness to manual palpation
  - ■ Nausea and vomiting does not occur in tension-type headache
  - ■ Individuals with tension-type headache do not have more than one of photophobia or phonophobia and if present, hypersensitivity to external stimuli is not prominent

■ Diagnosis

- The diagnosis of CTTH is based on operational diagnostic criteria (see Box 26.1)
- The differential diagnosis of CTTH includes chronic migraine (see Chapter 25), new daily persistent headache (see Chapter 28), cervicogenic headache (see Chapter 37), medication-overuse headache (see Chapter 35), and secondary causes of headache (see Chapters 29, 30, 31, 32, 33, 34, 35, 36, 37)
- Chronic migraine: The main difference between CTTH and chronic migraine is that individuals with chronic migraine have

Box 26.1 Chronic tension-type headache – International Headache Society diagnostic criteria

Diagnostic criteria:

A. Headache occurring on ≥15 days per month on average for >3 months (≥180 days per year) and fulfilling criteria B–D

B. Headache lasts hours or may be continuous

C. Headache has at least two of the following characteristics:
   1. bilateral location
   2. pressing/tightening (non-pulsating) quality
   3. mild or moderate intensity
   4. not aggravated by routine physical activity such as walking or climbing stairs

D. Both of the following:
   ■ no more than one of photophobia, phonophobia or mild nausea
   ■ neither moderate or severe nausea nor vomiting

E. Not attributed to another disorder

a history of episodic migraine which increased in frequency over time, transforming over months or years into a daily or near-daily headache. As the headaches become more frequent, some of the characteristic migraine features (nausea, vomiting, photophobia, and phonophobia) are lost. With chronic migraine, individuals frequently have days with headaches that resemble tension-type headache, but with other days on which headaches are migrainous.

● New daily persistent headache: The main difference between CTTH and new daily persistent headache is that with new daily persistent headache the headache begins and is daily within 72 hours; in contrast, CTTH usually evolves from episodic tension-type headache over weeks, months, or years

- Medication-overuse headache: This resembles CTTH. In the presence of medication overuse, a tentative diagnosis of probable tension-type headache and probable medication-overuse headache should be made. If headache persists after 2 months following withdrawal of the overused medication(s), than the diagnosis is CTTH. In contrast, if the headache resolves after withdrawal of the overused medication(s), the diagnosis should be coded as medication-overuse headache
- Cervicogenic headache: Like cervicogenic headache, tension-type headache may be most prominent in the occipitonuchal region; however, cervicogenic headache, unlike CTTH is a strictly unilateral disorder. Cervicogenic headache is a rare cause of headache and should be diagnosed cautiously and according to ICHD-2 classification (see Chapter 37)
- Tension-type headache is nondescript and featureless. It is notable that headaches secondary to space-occupying lesions such as brain tumors may present identical to tension-type headache. Correspondingly, all patients with subacute onset of CTTH warrant neuroimaging
- Neuroimaging (CT or MRI) is recommended if any "red flags" are identified on history or physical examination (see Table 24.2)

■ Treatment

- Treatment of tension-type headache includes lifestyle modifications to minimize headache occurrence, nonpharmacologic treatment modalities, and acute and prophylactic pharmacologic treatment
- An important early step in tension-type headache management is education about avoiding trigger factors and implementation of stress management and regular exercise programs to avoid/minimize tension-type headaches

- Use of over-the-counter analgesics such as acetaminophen, NSAIDs, or acetylsalicylic acid should be restricted to <15 days per month to avoid precipitation of medication-overuse headache. Use of combination products with caffeine or codeine should be restricted to <10 days per month to avoid precipitation of medication-overuse headache

- Non-pharmacologic therapy including biofeedback, cognitive-behavioral therapy, and relaxation therapy have been empirically validated as potentially efficacious treatments for CTTH. In some studies, the efficacy is as high as seen in studies on pharmacologic prophylactic therapy

- Prophylactic therapy is warranted when headaches are interfering with work, school, quality of life, and/or over-the-counter analgesic use is escalating (>10–15 days per month). There is some evidence to support use of the tricyclic antidepressants (i.e., amitriptyline or nortriptyline) and topiramate. Tricyclic antidepressants should be started at a low dose (10–25 mg orally every night) and increased gradually to the lowest effective and well-tolerated dose (may be 10–100 mg orally every night). Topiramate is typically started at 25 mg every night with a dose increase of 25 mg per week to a goal of 50–100 mg every night

- The is no solid evidence on which to advocate for the use of SSRIs, botulinum toxin type A, tizanidine, gabapentin, or any other pharmacologic prophylactic therapy for CTTH

- There may be a synergistic or additive effect from combining nonpharmacologic therapy (i.e., cognitive-behavioral therapy) and pharmacologic prophylactic therapy (i.e., tricyclic antidepressants)

- Manual therapies are hard to study in a randomized, placebo-controlled manner. There is some evidence to support the role of acupuncture and physical therapies (massage, physical therapy)

- There is little evidence to support the role of chiropractic manipulation, transcutaneous electrical nerve stimulation, oromandibular appliances, homeopathy, naturopathic treatments, and craniosacral therapy
- Comorbid psychiatric conditions such as depression should be appropriately addressed and managed

■ Outcome

- Avoidance of trigger factors, nonpharmacologic treatment interventions and/or pharmacologic prophylaxis with tricyclic antidepressants can help a significant proportion of individuals with CTTH

■ Further reading

Bigal ME, Lipton RB. Tension-type headache: classification and diagnosis. *Curr Pain Headache Rep* 2005;**9**:436–441.

Couch JR. The long-term prognosis of tension-type headache. *Curr Pain Headache Rep* 2005;**9**:423–429.

Holroyd KA, O'Donnell FJ, Stensland M, *et al*. Management of chronic tension-type headache with tricyclic antidepressant medication, stress management therapy, and their combination: a randomized, controlled trial. *JAMA* 2001;**285**:2208–2215.

Lanaerts ME. Pharmacoprophylaxis of tension-type headache. *Curr Pain Headache Rep* 2005;**9**:442–447.

Lenaerts ME. Burden of tension-type headache. *Curr Pain Headache Rep* 2006;**10**:459–462.

27

Hemicrania continua

■ Key points

- Hemicrania continua presents as a continuous, strictly unilateral headache with periodic exacerbations
- Patients have a complete response to adequate doses of indomethacin
- Brain imaging is recommended to investigate for secondary causes that can mimic the primary condition

■ General overview

- Hemicrania continua is one of the indomethacin-responsive headache syndromes
- It is characterized by unilateral head pain that is continuous but fluctuating in severity
- It may be accompanied by cranial autonomic features, migrainous features, jabs and jolts, and ocular discomfort
- It is more common in women than men (2:1)
- It may be precipitated by head trauma

■ Clinical features

- Headache
  - Continuous from onset in majority of patients, but may start as episodic attacks of prolonged unilateral headaches that last for days or weeks

- Unilateral without side-shift
- Mild to moderately severe intensity
- May be anterior and/or posteriorly located
  - Forehead, temple, orbit, occiput are the most common areas
- Dull, aching, or pressure
- Superimposed pain exacerbations
  - Occur on the same side as the continuous pain
  - Severe pain intensity
  - Throbbing or stabbing
- Associated features
  - Often associated with one or more of the following cranial autonomic features, although not as prominent as that seen with cluster headache:
    - Tearing – most common
    - Conjunctival injection
    - Nasal congestion
    - Rhinorrhea
    - Ptosis
    - Eyelid edema
    - Miosis
  - Exacerbations may be associated with migrainous features:
    - Photophobia
    - Phonophobia
    - Nausea
    - Vomiting
  - Duration lasts between hours to days
  - Ocular discomfort – often described as a feeling of sand in the eye
- Jabs and jolts
  - Also known as idiopathic stabbing headache or ice-pick pain
  - Brief (1–2 seconds), sharp, stabs of pain, often ipsilateral to the headache

■ Diagnosis

- The diagnosis of hemicrania continua is based on operational diagnostic criteria (Box 27.1)
- Physical exam
  - During exacerbation, ≥1 cranial autonomic features may be observed
    - Lacrimation
    - Conjunctival injection
    - Rhinorrhea
    - Ptosis
    - Eyelid edema
    - Miosis
  - Contrast and noncontrast brain MRI
    - Recommended to exclude secondary causes (mimics)

Box 27.1 Hemicrania continua – International Headache Society diagnostic criteria

A. Headache for >3 months fulfilling criteria B–D
B. All of the following characteristics:
  1. unilateral pain without side-shift
  2. daily and continuous, without pain-free periods
  3. moderate intensity, but with exacerbations of severe pain
C. At least one of the following autonomic features occurs during exacerbations and ipsilateral to the side of pain:
  1. conjunctival injection and/or lacrimation
  2. nasal congestion and/or rhinorrhea
  3. ptosis and/or miosis
D. Complete response to therapeutic doses of indomethacin
E. Not attributed to another disorder

- Several cases have been described:
  - Sphenoid sinusitis
  - Sphenoid tumor
  - Internal carotid artery dissection – if suspected, would require further imaging of the intra/extracranial arteries
  - Stroke
  - Prolactinoma
- Secondary cases not excluded by brain MRI
  - Lung malignancy (Pancoast tumor)
  - HIV infection

■ Treatment

- By definition, hemicrania continua is completely responsive to indomethacin
  - Patients with suspected hemicrania continua may be prescribed an "indomethacin trial." An example of such a treatment trial is:
    - 25 mg orally three times daily × 3 days, then
    - 50 mg orally three times daily × 3 days, then
    - 75 mg orally three times daily × 3 days
  - If resolution of headache occurs, patients are instructed to continue taking that dose of indomethacin for a period of days to weeks and then a gradual taper by 25 mg every 3 days is initiated until the lowest effective dose is achieved
    - Once the lowest effective dose is determined, sustained-release indomethacin may be prescribed
    - Patients may require treatment with a gastric mucosal protective agent (such as a proton-pump inhibitor) during indomethacin therapy due to gastrointestinal toxicity

- Indomethacin dose should be slowly tapered or discontinued approximately every 3 months in order to determine if continued treatment is necessary
  - Some patients will not have headache recurrence
- Some patients with a classical clinical picture of hemicrania continua do not respond to indomethacin, while in others, the effectiveness of indomethacin might wane
- Some patients will not tolerate indomethacin side-effects
- Other therapies
  - Cyclooxygenase-2 inhibitors
  - Other NSAIDs (e.g., sulindac)
  - Occipital nerve block
  - Corticosteroids
  - Gabapentin
  - Methysergide
  - Lithium
  - Lamotrigine
  - Dihydroergotamine
  - Melatonin
  - Occipital nerve stimulation

■ Outcome

- Some patients will have remission and will be able to discontinue therapy
- Others will require long-term therapy

■ Further reading

Boes CJ, Swanson JW. Paroxysmal hemicrania, SUNCT, and hemicrania continua. *Semin Neurol* 2006;**26**:260–270.

Pareja JA, Vincent M, Antonaci F, Sjaastad O. Hemicrania continua: diagnostic criteria and nosologic status. *Cephalalgia* 2001;**21**:874–877.

Rapoport AM, Bigal ME. Hemicrania continua: clinical and nosographic update. *Neurol Sci* 2003;**24**:S118–S121.

Silberstein SD, Peres MFP. Hemicrania continua. *Arch Neurol* 2002;**59**:1029–1030.

Trucco M, Mainardi F, Maggioni F, *et al*. Chronic paroxysmal hemicrania, hemicrania continua and SUNCT syndrome in association with other pathologies: a review. *Cephalalgia* 2004;**24**:173–184.

28

New daily persistent headache

■ Key points

- A primary headache disorder characterized by the subacute onset (over 72 hours) of a daily, unremitting headache
- The headache may resemble chronic tension-type headache (CTTH) or chronic migraine, however, unlike both of these, which usually evolve over weeks or months from an episodic headache disorder, new daily persistent headache (NDPH) begins rather abruptly
- NDPH is a diagnosis of exclusion; thorough neuroimaging and a hematologic workup are required to exclude secondary causes
- The headache may resolve on its own *or* be highly refractory to treatment

■ General overview

- An uncommon primary headache syndrome recently included in ICHD-2
- Most common in adolescents and young adults
- Epidemiology unknown; occurs in up to 10% of patients in tertiary headache clinics
- Underlying etiology is unknown; up to 30% in one study reported a recent infection or flulike illness at the time of headache onset

- There are two clinical subtypes – a benign self-limited form and a refractory form resistant to aggressive therapy

■ Clinical features

- Headache
  - Typically bilateral
  - Pain is usually continuous
  - Intensity is usually moderate but can be mild or severe
  - Pain may be described as pressure or tightening; throbbing/pulsating has been described although is excluded in the ICHD-2 diagnostic criteria
  - Pain may be aggravated by physical activity/exercise
- Associated features
  - "Migrainous" features (nausea, vomiting, phono/photophobia) can occur but are typically not the most prominent symptoms
  - No associated trigeminal autonomic features (e.g., lacrimation, conjunctival injection)
  - No associated systemic or neurologic symptoms

■ Diagnosis

- The diagnosis of NDPH is based on operational diagnostic criteria (see Box 28.1)
- The differential diagnosis of NDPH includes CTTH (see Chapter 26), chronic migraine (see Chapter 25), and secondary causes of chronic headaches (see Chapters 29, 30, 31, 32, 33, 34, 35, 36, 37)
- CTTH: The main difference between NDPH and CTTH is that the latter evolves from escalating episodic tension-type headaches whereas NDPH evolves over <72 hours without a history of previous escalating headache

Box 28.1 New daily persistent headache – International Headache Society diagnostic criteria

Diagnostic criteria:

A. Headache that, within 3 days of onset, fulfils criteria B–D

B. Headache is present daily, and is unremitting, for >3 months

C. At least two of the following pain characteristics:
   1. bilateral location
   2. pressing/tightening (non-pulsating) quality
   3. mild or moderate intensity
   4. not aggravated by routine physical activity such as walking or climbing

D. Both of the following:
   1. no more than one of photophobia, phonophobia or mild nausea
   2. neither moderate or severe nausea nor vomiting

E. Not attributed to another disorder

- Chronic migraine: The main difference between NDPH and chronic migraine is the absence of an escalating history of episodic migraine and/or the absence of prominent migrainous features in NDPH
- The headache observed in spontaneous intracranial hypotension can resemble NDPH *if* the headaches loses its characteristic positional component over time and/or *if* the presence of a positional component was overlooked on history
- NDPH is a diagnosis of exclusion and secondary causes of CDH must be excluded
  - Blood tests
    - Complete blood count (to rule out chronic anemia or chronic infection), thyroid-stimulating hormone (TSH) (to rule out hypothyroidism); C-reactive protein and erythrocyte sedimentation rate (ESR) in patients over the age of 50 years

- MRI brain
  - To rule out space-occupying lesion, hydrocephalus
  - With gadolinium – to rule out spontaneous intracranial hypotension
  - ± MR venography – to rule out cerebral venous sinus thrombosis
- Lumbar puncture
  - To exclude disorders of increased cerebrospinal fluid (CSF) pressure (idiopathic intracranial hypertension), decreased CSF pressure (spontaneous intracranial hypotension), or chronic infection (chronic meningitis)

■ Treatment

- There is no known consistently effective acute or prophylactic therapy. Standard acute and prophylactic therapies for CTTH and chronic migraine headache could be tried on a trial-and-error basis and therapeutic options rotated until an effective treatment is found
- Caution should be exercised to avoid developing concomitant medication-overuse headache

■ Outcome

- There are two clinical subtypes of NDPH
  - A benign, self-limited syndrome that resolves on its own with or without medical consultation or intervention
  - A highly refractory subtype resistant to traditional nonpharmacologic and pharmacologic acute and prophylactic therapies for chronic headache

■ Further reading

Bigal ME, Lipton RB, Tepper SJ, *et al*. Primary chronic daily headache and its subtypes in adolescents and adults. *Neurology* 2004;**63**:843–847.

Diaz-Mitoma F, Vanast WJ, Tyrrell DL. Increased frequency of Epstein–Barr virus excretion in patients with new daily persistent headaches. *Lancet* 1987;**21**:411–415.

Evans RW. New daily persistent headache. *Curr Pain Headache Rep* 2003;**7**:303–307.

Kung E, Tepper SJ, Rapoport AM, *et al*. New daily persistent headache in the paediatric population. *Cephalalgia* 2009;**29**:17–22.

Mack KJ. New daily persistent headache in children and adults. *Curr Pain Headache Rep* 2009;**13**:47–51.

Meineri P, Torre E, Rota E, *et al*. New daily persistent headache: clinical and serological characteristics in a retrospective study. *Neurol Sci* 2004;**25** (Suppl 3):S281–S282.

Rozen TD. New daily persistent headache. *Curr Pain Headache Rep* 2003;**7**:218–223.

Takase Y, Nakano M, Tatsumi C, *et al*. Clinical features, effectiveness of drug-based treatment, and prognosis of new daily persistent headache (NDPH): 30 cases in Japan. *Cephalalgia* 2004;**24**:955–959.

Vanast WJ. New daily persistent headaches: definition of a benign syndrome. *Headache* 1986;**26**:317.

Vanast WJ, Diaz-Mitoma F, Tyrrell DL. Hypothesis: chronic benign daily headache is an immune disorder with a viral trigger. *Headache* 1987;**27**:138–142.

29

Giant cell arteritis

■ Key points

- Giant cell arteritis (GCA) is a vasculitis of the medium and large arteries that preferentially affects individuals over 50 years
- It classically presents with new-onset persistent headache, abnormal temporal artery, and elevated serum inflammatory markers; 2%–10% of patients have a normal erythrocyte sedimentation rate
- Histologic confirmation via temporal artery biopsy is the gold standard for the diagnosis of GCA
- Corticosteroid treatment should be initiated immediately when GCA is suspected, and should not be delayed while awaiting biopsy
- Long-term treatment with corticosteroids is often required; 40%–45% still require treatment at 5 years while 25% still require treatment at 9 years

■ General overview

- GCA is also known as temporal arteritis and Horton disease
- GCA involves medium and large arteries, with a predilection for those originating from the arch of the aorta
- Most commonly affects those 50 years or older with an increasing incidence with advancing age
- Females are affected more commonly than males (approximately 3:1)

■ Clinical features (Box 29.1)

- Headache
  - 90% of patients have headache during the course of the disease
  - 50% of patients present with headache
  - Suspect GCA in all patients 50 years or older with new-onset headache or a significant change in their prior headache pattern
  - Headache characteristics and location may be quite variable and may resemble primary headache disorders
- Temporal artery tenderness
- Claudication
  - 30%–70% have claudication
  - Jaw, tongue, limb, swallowing
- Polymyalgia rheumatica
  - 35%–50% of patients with GCA have polymyalgia rheumatica
  - 15%–20% of patients with polymyalgia rheumatica have GCA
  - Pain and stiffness in the neck, shoulders, and pelvic girdle

Box 29.1 Clinical manifestations of giant cell arteritis

- Headache
- Claudication (jaw, tongue, limb, swallowing)
- Systemic manifestations (fever, weight loss, sweats, malaise)
- Polymyalgia rheumatica
- Neuroophthalmologic (acute ischemic optic neuropathy, amaurosis fugax)
- Large artery involvement (aortic dissection, aortic aneurysm, arterial stenosis)
- Temporal artery tenderness
- Neuropathy
- Stroke/transient ischemic attack (TIA)

- Systemic symptoms
  - Malaise
  - Fever
  - Weight loss
  - Night sweats (50% of patients)
- Neuroophthalmologic
  - Amaurosis fugax – 10% of GCA patients
  - Acute ischemic optic neuropathy – 10%–30%
    - Most commonly manifests as a permanent altitudinal visual field cut
    - Secondary to posterior ciliary arteritis
    - Corticosteroids decrease the risk of contralateral eye involvement
- Large artery complications
  - 25% of patients
  - May be present at time of diagnosis but more often present years later
  - Aortic dissection, aortic aneurysm, large artery stenosis
- Other clinical features
  - 15% have mononeuropathy or peripheral neuropathy
  - 7% have a TIA or stroke

■ Diagnosis (Box 29.2)

- Physical exam
  - Temporal artery
    - Loss of pulse
    - Nodularity
    - Tenderness to palpation
  - Fever
- Laboratory exam
  - ESR

> **Box 29.2 Giant cell arteritis – American College of Rheumatology diagnostic criteria**
>
> Three or more of the following five criteria must be present:
> 1. Age at disease onset ≥50 years
> 2. New headache
> 3. Temporal artery abnormality (tenderness to palpation or decreased pulsation)
> 4. Erythrocyte sedimentation rate ≥50 mm/hour by the Westergren method
> 5. Abnormal temporal artery biopsy (vasculitis characterized by predominance of mononuclear cell infiltration or granulomatous inflammation, usually with multinucleated giant cells)

- 47–107 mm/hour – doubles the odds of positive biopsy
- >107 mm/hour – 2.7 odds of positive biopsy
- 2%–10% of patients with GCA have a normal ESR
- C-reactive protein
  - >2.45 mg/dL – 3.2 odds of positive biopsy
- Anemia
- Thrombocytosis
- Temporal artery biopsy
  - New-onset headache, claudication, abnormal temporal artery on exam, and systemic symptoms have consistently been associated with positive likelihood ratios for GCA on temporal artery biopsy
  - At least 20 mm section, with histologic examination at multiple sites
  - At our institution, a 3–4 cm biopsy is taken from the temporal artery most likely involved. Frozen section analysis is performed

and if negative, a biopsy is taken from the contralateral artery. Permanent sections of both samples are examined

■ 10%–15% of patients with GCA have negative biopsies, most probably due to "skip lesions" or characteristic areas of involvement interspersed with normal arterial tissues

■ Treatment

- Corticosteroids are the mainstay of treatment
  - ■ Should be initiated immediately when GCA is suspected (see Fig. 29.1)
    - Treatment should not be delayed while awaiting biopsy
    - Biopsy should be undertaken within 2 weeks of corticosteroid initiation

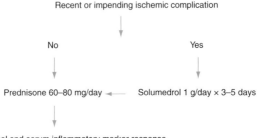

Recent or impending ischemic complication

No → Prednisone 60–80 mg/day ← Yes → Solumedrol 1 g/day × 3–5 days

Clinical and serum inflammatory marker response

No → Increase prednisone to 1.5–2.0 mg/kg per day

Yes → Continue same dose for 2–4 weeks then decrease by 10 mg daily each 2 weeks until reaching 40 mg/day. Then decrease by no more than 10% of daily dose every 2 weeks while monitoring symptoms and inflammatory markers.

Fig. 29.1 Treatment of giant cell arteritis.

- Small studies suggest that although histologic changes may occur, biopsy results are not significantly altered by up to 6 weeks of prior corticosteroid therapy
- Resolution of headache and systemic symptoms and normalization of serum inflammatory markers is expected
- Symptoms and inflammatory markers (especially ESR and C-reactive protein [CRP]) are used as indicators of disease activity and are monitored during corticosteroid taper
- Although side-effects of long-term corticosteroid use are common, the efficacy of steroid-sparing agents is not proven and their use cannot be recommended at this time

■ Outcome

- Relapse most commonly occurs within the first month of corticosteroid withdrawal but relapse rates are elevated for the first year
- Recurrence is rare when daily doses remain at 7.5 mg or higher
- Many patients require prolonged corticosteroid treatment when tapering attempts fail
  - 40%–45% still require treatment at 5 years
  - 25% still require treatment at 9 years

■ Further reading

Caselli RJ, Hunder GG, Whisnant JP. Neurologic disease in biopsy-proven giant cell (temporal) arteritis. *Neurology* 1988;**38**:352–359.

Gonzalez-Gay MA, Barcia-Porrua C, Llorca J, *et al.* Biopsy-negative giant cell arteritis: clinical spectrum and predictive factors for positive temporal artery biopsy. *Semin Arthritis Rheum* 2001;**30**:249–256.

Hayreh SS, Podhajsky PA, Raman R, Zimmerman B. Giant cell arteritis: validity and reliability of various diagnostic criteria. *Am J Ophthal* 1997;**123**:285–296.

Hunder GG, Bloch DA, Michel BA, *et al.* The American College of Rheumatology 1990 criteria for the classification of giant cell arteritis. *Arthritis Rheum* 1990;**33**:1122–1128.

Huston KA, Hunder GG, Lie JT. Temporal arteritis: a 25-year epidemiologic, clinical, and pathologic study. *Ann Intern Med* 1978;**88**:162–167.

30

Cerebral venous sinus thrombosis

■ Key points

- The majority of patients with cerebral venous sinus thrombosis (CVST) experience headaches
- In most patients, the headache occurs in association with other signs and symptoms such as papilledema, focal neurologic symptoms and signs, seizures, or altered level of consciousness
- A minority of patients with cerebral venous sinus thrombosis present with isolated headaches
- Venous obstruction may result in cerebral edema and cerebral infarctions
- Outcome is improved by early diagnosis and management

■ General overview

- CVST refers to the occlusion of one or more of the draining veins or sinuses of the brain (Fig. 30.1)
- Although once considered a rare disorder, modern imaging techniques have allowed for an increased likelihood of diagnosis
- The clinical manifestations of CVST and outcomes of patients with CVST vary widely
- Headache is the most frequent symptom of CVST

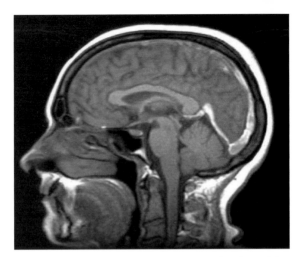

Fig. 30.1 Sagittal T1-weighted MRI brain demonstrating thrombosis of the superior sagittal and straight cerebral sinuses.

- CVST more commonly occurs in patients with risk factors for thromboembolic disease:
  - The puerperium
  - Hematologic disorders
  - Presence of prothrombotic factors
  - Oral contraceptive use
  - Dehydration
  - Cancer
  - Personal or family history of venous thromboembolic disease

■ Clinical features

- Most patients present with headache in association with focal neurologic symptoms and signs or seizures

- A minority of patients may present with isolated headache, isolated intracranial hypertension, subacute encephalopathy, or the syndrome of septic cavernous sinus thrombosis
- Headache
  - Present in at least 80% of patients
    - Most common initial symptom
  - Up to ⅓ of patients present with headache without other symptoms
  - Onset is often subacute and gradually progressive over a few days
  - <10% of patients present with "thunderclap headache"
  - May present as new daily persistent headache or chronic daily headache
  - Most often persistent but may be intermittent
  - Severity and localization vary (mild to severe; localized to diffuse)
  - Pain is exacerbated by increases in intracranial pressure
    - Coughing
    - Sneezing
    - Valsalva
    - Supine position – headaches may be worse upon awakening in the morning
    - Stooping
- Focal deficits and/or seizures
  - Aphasia/dysphasia
  - Hemiplegia
  - Visuospatial disorders
  - Hemianopia
  - Amnesia
  - Generalized seizures
  - Focal seizures

- Isolated intracranial hypertension
  - Headache
  - Papilledema
  - Sixth nerve palsy (diplopia)
  - Mimics pseudotumor cerebri (idiopathic intracranial hypertension)
- Subacute encephalopathy
  - Altered mental status
  - Seizures
- Cavernous sinus thrombosis
  - Cavernous sinus contains
    - Oculomotor nerve (cranial nerve III)
    - Trochlear nerve (cranial nerve IV)
    - First two branches of the trigeminal nerve (cranial nerves V1 and V2)
    - Abducens nerve (cranial nerve VI)
  - Most commonly manifests as:
    - Headache
    - Painful cranial nerve III or IV palsy (diplopia)
    - Periorbital edema
    - Fever
  - May be secondary to infections involving the face, sphenoid and ethmoid sinuses, dental infections, or mastoiditis
  - Often spreads, resulting in bilateral involvement

■ Diagnosis

- Physical exam
  - Papilledema
  - Focal neurologic deficits
  - Cavernous sinus thrombosis
    - Fever
    - Periorbital edema

- Ptosis
- Proptosis
- Chemosis
- Ocular muscle paralysis
- Mydriasis
- Facial hypo- or hyperesthesia
- Depressed mental status
- Imaging
  - CT brain
    - Low sensitivity and specificity
    - Thrombosed venous sinus and cortical veins
    - Homogeneous hyperdensity
      - Empty delta sign
      - Dense vein sign
      - Cord sign
      - Edema – cerebral infarctions
      - Venous infarctions (venous hypertension); location depends on cortical vein or venous sinus that is thrombosed
      - May be bilateral, especially in case of sagittal sinus thrombosis with bilateral parasagittal parietal vertex infarctions
    - Hemorrhage
      - Most commonly small petechial hemorrhages from venous infarction
      - May be bilateral
      - Uncommonly, large subcortical hematoma
  - MRI brain
    - Edema
      - Hyperintense on T2-weighted images
      - Typically subcortical but may involve the cortex
      - May be bilateral

- Hemorrhage
  - Venous infarction
  - Hypointense on T2-weighted images in the early stages
- Most commonly small petechial hemorrhages, but may be a large subcortical hematoma
  - Does not conform to a major arterial territory
  - May be bilateral
- Thrombosed venous sinus
  - Replacement of the venous sinus flow void with increased signal intensity of the thrombus (see Fig 30.1)
- Cavernous sinus thrombosis
  - Orbital MRI with gadolinium
  - Areas of irregular enhancement in the cavernous sinus
  - Thickened lateral walls
  - Sinus bulging
  - MRV brain
    - Signal dropout in the thrombosed venous sinus
    - Must be differentiated from a congenitally small nonoccluded venous sinus
    - Asymmetry of the venous sinuses is common
  - Conventional angiography
    - May be necessary if other imaging studies are contraindicated or if diagnostic uncertainty remains
- Lumbar puncture
  - Elevated opening pressure
    - May be the only lumbar puncture abnormality in 40% of patients
  - Lymphocytic pleocytosis
  - Elevated red blood cell count
  - Elevated protein levels

- Cavernous sinus thrombosis
  - Inflammatory spinal fluid – most common
  - Lymphocytosis with normal glucose, protein, culture negative
  - Lymphocytosis with low glucose, high protein, culture positive

Treatment

- Anticoagulation
  - Treatment of choice
  - Reduces risk of venous infarction, neurologic worsening, and pulmonary embolism
  - Increases risk of hemorrhage
- Thrombolysis
  - May be indicated in patients whose condition worsens despite anticoagulation, or in patients with an absolute contraindication to heparin or warfarin anticoagulation
    - Targeted infusion of thrombolytics
    - Mechanical disruption of thrombus
- Septic cavernous sinus thrombosis
  - High-dose intravenous antibiotics
  - Anticoagulation
  - Corticosteroids
  - Surgical intervention
    - Not commonly required

Outcome

- Varies widely from complete resolution of symptoms to permanent deficits or death due to stroke and cerebral edema
  - Mortality rate is 5%–15%
  - Possible indicators of poor prognosis are:
    - Old age
    - Coma

- Deep venous system involvement
- Significant elevations of intracranial pressure
- Infectious or malignant causes
- Hemorrhagic infarcts
- Uncontrolled seizures
- Pulmonary embolism
- Complete recovery occurs in 35%–85% of patients

■ Further reading

Agostini E. Headache in cerebral venous thrombosis. *Neurol Sci* 2004;**25**: S206–S210.

Bousser MG. Cerebral venous thrombosis: diagnosis and management. *J Neurol* 2000;**247**:252–258.

Connor SEJ, Jarosz JM. Magnetic resonance imaging of cerebral venous sinus thrombosis. *Clin Radiol* 2002;**57**:449–461.

Cumurciuc R, Crassard I, Sarov M, *et al*. Headache as the only neurological sign of cerebral venous thrombosis: a series of 17 cases. *J Neurol Neurosurg Psychiatry* 2005;**76**:1084–1087.

de Bruijn SFTM, de Haan RJ, Stam J, for the Cerebral Venous Sinus Thrombosis Study Group. Clinical features and prognostic factors of cerebral venous sinus thrombosis in a prospective series of 59 patients. *J Neurol Neurosurg Psychiatry* 2001;**70**:105–108.

de Bruijn SFTM, Stam J, Kappelle LJ, for CVST Study Group. Thunderclap headache as first symptom of cerebral venous sinus thrombosis. *Lancet* 1996;**348**:1623–1625.

Ebright JR, Pace MT, Niazi AF. Septic thrombosis of the cavernous sinus. *Arch Intern Med* 2001;**161**:2671–2676.

Stam J, de Bruijn SFTM, DeVeber G. Anticoagulation for cerebral sinus thrombosis. *Cochrane Database Syst Rev* 2002;**4**:CD002005.

Terazzi E, Mittino D, Ruda R, Cerrato P, *et al*. Cerebral venous thrombosis: a retrospective multicentre study of 48 patients. *Neurol Sci* 2005;**25**: 311–315.

31

Spontaneous intracranial hypotension

■ Key points

- Spontaneous intracranial hypotension (SIH) classically presents with headache, low CSF pressure, and MR enhancement of the pachymeninges, i.e., the dura
- The typical headache is holocephalic, bilateral and worse when upright
- Patients with SIH need detailed investigation and referral for expert opinion given the difficulty in finding and treating the putative CSF leak

■ General overview

- Usually no definite history of any event that directly relates to the onset of symptoms, such as would occur in patients with post-lumbar puncture headache. Some patients report a trivial trauma that precedes onset of symptoms (see Box 31.1)
- The classical orthostatic headache may or may not be present and chronic headache can occur over time in some patients, with rare cases with no headache

Box 31.1 Etiology of SIH (after Mokri, 2004)

- Unknown cause (common)
- Weakness of dural sac due to meningeal diverticula or abnormal connective tissue
- Dural tear from spondylosis or disk herniation
- Trivial trauma

■ Clinical features

- Headache
  - No typical headache features in terms of quality or severity
    - Patients might have a background history of a primary headache
    - Holocephalic headache with or without throbbing may occur
  - Most patients have more severe pain when upright and relief with lying down. Not all patients have positional headaches
  - Although most patients with orthostatic headaches have worsening of headache intensity within minutes of becoming upright, in some patients worsening occurs only after being upright for hours
  - Rarely, patients with SIH have worse headaches when lying and improvement with standing
  - May mimic primary headache disorders such as tension-type headache and migraine
  - Occurs daily and interferes with life activities
- Other clinical features
  - Diplopia, blurring of vision, field cut, or photophobia may occur

- Cranial nerve abnormalities rare but cranial nerves III and IV can be involved
- Facial numbness or weakness can occur
- Dizziness and interscapular, cervical, or low back pain
- Encephalopathy or altered states of consciousness have also been reported

■ Diagnosis

- The diagnosis of SIH depends on: a careful inquiry of the history, particularly directed towards positional and diurnal changes in headache; a careful physical and neurologic examination; and cerebral imaging sufficient to make the diagnosis, along with CSF pressure measurement if needed
- History
  - See Boxes 31.2 and 31.3 for criteria and Box 31.1 for the risk factors
- Neurological exam
  - Usually normal
  - No papilledema

Box 31.2 Spontaneous intracranial hypotension – clinical features

- Headache worse when upright and relieved by lying down
- Occasionally paradoxical headache, better lying than when upright
- Hard to diagnose and many self-limited
- Typically requires diagnosis and management by a specialist. Appropriate therapy can be curative in some patients

Box 31.3 Spontaneous intracranial hypotension, primary intracranial hypotension, low-CSF volume headache – International Headache Society diagnostic criteria

Diagnostic criteria:

A. Diffuse and/or dull headache that worsens within 15 minutes after sitting or standing, with at least one of the following and fulfilling criterion D:
   1. neck stiffness
   2. tinnitus
   3. hypacusia
   4. photophobia
   5. nausea
B. At least one of the following:
   1. evidence of low CSF pressure on MRI (*eg*, pachymeningeal enhancement)
   2. evidence of CSF leakage on conventional myelography, CT myelography or cisternography
   3. CSF opening pressure <60 mm H_2O in sitting position
C. No history of dural puncture or other cause of CSF fistula
D. Headache resolves within 72 hours after epidural blood patching

- Lumbar puncture
  - Opening pressure usually low, but results inconsistent
  - Clear or xanthochromic fluid, with or without white or red blood cell pleocytosis
  - Protein levels may be high or normal
- Imaging
  - Unless contraindicated, MRI with gadolinium is the initial imaging modality of choice as it is superior to CT with contrast in identifying and characterizing SIH (Fig. 31.1)

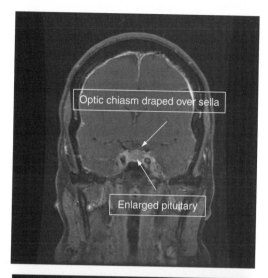

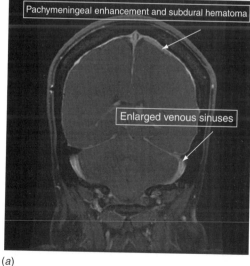

(*a*)

Fig. 31.1 (*a–c*) Magnetic resonance imaging features of cerebrospinal fluid leak and intracranial hypotension.

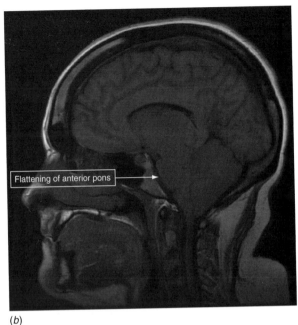

Flattening of anterior pons

(b)

Fig. 31.1 (cont.)

- Diffuse enhancement of dura or pachymeninges, rarely absent
- Sagging brain and crowded brain stem, which may mimic Chiari I malformation
- Subdural fluid collections and engorged venous sinuses
- Optic nerves flattened
- Enlarged pituitary
- Extra-arachnoid fluid and sometimes diverticula or the level of leak are seen in the spine

■ CT
  - Can be done if MRI is contraindicated or prior to lumbar puncture
  - May detect subdural collection or tentorial enhancement

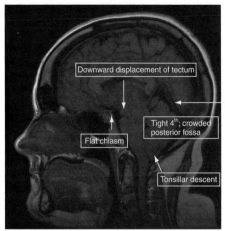

(c)

Fig. 31.1 (cont.)

- ▪ Radioisotope cisternography
  - ● May show site of leak or basal accumulation of radioisotope
- ▪ CT myelogram
  - ● May detect site of CSF leak

■ Treatment

- ● Conservative measures
  - ▪ Bed rest
  - ▪ Hydration
  - ▪ Abdominal binders
  - ▪ Trendelenburg position
- ● Medications
  - ▪ Try caffeine, aminophylline (anecdotal)
  - ▪ Steroids (unproven)
  - ▪ Analgesics

- Epidural blood patches
  - Lumbar, then thoracic and cervical if necessary
  - Other CSF patching procedures
- Surgery
  - Repair of defect causing the leak, if it can be found
  - There may be more than one leak

■ Further reading

Headache Classification Subcommittee of the International Headache Society. The International Classification of Headache Disorders, 2nd edn. *Cephalalgia* 2004;**24**(Suppl 1):9–160.

Miyazawa K, Shiga Y, Hasegawa T, *et al*. CSF hypovolemia vs intracranial hypotension in "spontaneous intracranial hypotension syndrome." *Neurology* 2003;**60**:941–947.

Mokri B. Spontaneous cerebrospinal fluid leaks: from intracranial hypotension to cerebrospinal fluid hypovolemia-evolution of a concept. *Mayo Clin Proc* 1999;**74**:1113–1123.

Mokri B. The Monro-Kellie hypothesis. Applications in CSF volume depletion. *Neurology* 2001;**56**:1746–1748.

Mokri B. Low cerebrospinal fluid pressure syndromes. *Neurol Clin* 2004;**22**:55–7.

Mokri B, Aksamit AJ, Atkinson JLD. Paradoxical postural headaches in cerebrospinal fluid leaks. *Cephalalgia* 2004;**24**:883–887.

Mokri B, Atkinson JLD, Dodick DW, *et al.* Absent pachymeningeal gadolinium enhancement on cranial MRI despite symptomatic CSF leak. *Neurology* 1999;**53**:402–404.

Mokri B, Atkinson JLD, Piepgras DG. Absent headaches despite CSF volume depletion (intracranial hypotension). *Neurology* 2000;**55**:1722–1724.

Schievink WI. Spontaneous spinal cerebrospinal fluid leaks and intracranial hypotension. *JAMA* 2006;**295**:2286–2296.

Vilming ST, Mokri B. Low cerebrospinal fluid pressure. In: Olesen J, Goadsby PJ, Ramadan NM *et al.*, eds. *The Headaches* 3rd edn, Philadelphia: PA: Lippincott Williams & Wilkins, 2006:935–943.

32

Idiopathic intracranial hypertension

■ Key points

- Idiopathic intracranial hypertension (IHH; pseudotumor cerebri) is characterized by elevated intracranial pressure without ventriculomegaly or mass lesion
- The disorder is most common in obese women younger than 45 years
- Headache is present in 95% of patients and has no particular distinguishing characteristics
- Pulsatile tinnitus and transient visual obscurations are common initial symptoms
- Diagnosis requires neuroimaging (MRI brain), lumbar puncture with opening pressure, CSF examination, and exclusion of secondary causes. Evaluation must include ophthalmologic examination with visual perimetry
- Prompt recognition and treatment is important to prevent visual loss
- There are both medical and surgical treatments – the goal of treatment is preservation of vision

■ General overview

- IIH occurs in individuals under 50 years, and most commonly in obese women of childbearing age

- Risk factors for IIH include:
  - Female sex
  - High body mass index (BMI >30)
  - Weight gain in the year prior to onset of symptoms (5%–15% of body weight)
  - Use of tetracycline antibiotics in the 6 months prior to onset of symptoms

■ Clinical features

SYMPTOMS

- Headache
  - Most common symptom (>90%)
  - No typical headache features in terms of quality or severity
  - Most often daily and progressive, although clinical features may mimic migraine
- Other relatively common symptoms
  - Transient visual obscurations (>75%)
    - Consists of partial or complete visual loss
    - May be unilateral or bilateral
    - Often provoked by changes in position or posture or Valsalva
    - Lasts <60 seconds
    - Not predictive of visual loss
  - Pulsatile tinnitus (>50%)
  - Diplopia
  - Partial visual field loss
  - Blurred vision

SIGNS

- Papilledema is the hallmark of IIH (Fig. 32.1), and is usually bilateral but may be asymmetric or unilateral

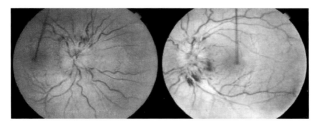

Fig. 32.1 Fundus images illustrating stage 5 papilledema. There is obscuration of the optic disk margins and vessels over the optic nerve, with flame-shaped hemorrhages and swelling of the optic nerve heads.

- Spontaneous venous pulsations (SVPs) usually indicate intracranial pressure <250 mm H_2O, but SVPs may be present when intracranial pressure is elevated
  - 25% of the normal population do not have SVPs, so their absence does not necessarily indicate elevated pressures
- Visual field defects
  - Usually inferonasal loss
  - Generalized constriction of visual field
  - Enlargement of physiologic blind spot
- Unilateral or bilateral lateral rectus palsy (false localizing abducens nerve palsy)

■ Diagnosis

- The critical elements of the diagnosis are:
  - Symptoms and signs consistent with and caused by raised intracranial pressure and papilledema
  - Elevated opening pressure ([OP] >250 mm H_2O) by lumbar puncture (**Note**: CSF pressure *must* be measured *only* in lateral decubitus position with legs partially extended and patient relaxed; if lumbar puncture done in sitting position or under fluoroscopy, patient must be moved into lateral decubitus position)

- OP between 200 mm H_2O and 250 mm H_2O is indeterminate
- OP >100 mm H_2O in children <8 years is abnormal
- OP >200 mm H_2O in children between 8 and 12 years is abnormal
- Normal CSF analysis
- Normal MRI brain with gadolinium and magnetic resonance venography (MRV)
  - MRI brain *must exclude* enlarged ventricles, mass lesion, and meningeal enhancement. MRV should exclude venous sinus thrombosis and transverse venous sinus stenosis
  - MRI may show empty sella turcica, distention of optic nerve sheaths, flattening of the posterior sclera, protrusion of optic nerve papillae into vitreous
  - MRV should exclude venous sinus thrombosis. It may show transverse sinus stenosis (TSS), which is usually a result of elevated intracranial pressure and resolves with effective treatment. Stenting of a TSS in patients unresponsive to medical management has led to a reduction in venous sinus pressure, intracranial pressure, and resolution of papilledema, headache, and other associated symptoms
- Ophthalmologic assessment
  - Best corrected visual acuity
  - Quantitative visual field testing by automated or kinetic (Goldman) perimetry
  - Intraocular pressure measurement
  - Stereoscopic evaluation of optic nerve and fundi
- Normal mental status and neurologic examination
- No secondary cause is identified (see Box 32.1)

Box 32.1 Disorders associated with idiopathic intracranial hypertension

Endocrine

- Obesity, recent weight gain
- Polycystic ovarian syndrome
- Addison disease
- Hypoparathyroidism
- Hyperthyroidism
- Orthostatic edema

Drugs and supplements

- Corticosteroids/corticosteroid withdrawal
- Vitamin A
- Accutane, *trans*-retinoic acid
- Tetracycline, minocycline, doxycycline
- Sulfa antibiotics
- Nalidixic acid
- Lithium carbonate
- Levothyroxine
- Luteinizing hormone-releasing hormone analog; growth hormone

Cerebral venous pressure elevation

- Cerebral venous sinus thrombosis
- Cerebral venous sinus stenosis
- Dural arteriovenous fistula
- Increased right heart pressure, superior vena cava syndrome

Other

- Antiphospholipid antibody syndrome
- Systemic lupus erythematosus
- Chronic obstructive pulmonary disease
- Renal failure
- Sleep apnea

■ Treatment

The primary objective of treatment is to preserve vision. Management of the headache may require a separate strategy. Longitudinal assessment of quantitative visual fields and visual acuity should guide treatment. There are no randomized controlled trials for any medical or surgical therapy for IIH.

MEDICAL TREATMENT

- Discontinue any offending medication or supplement
- Weight loss in obese patients
- Salt restriction
- Avoid corticosteroids
- Acetazolamide 1–2 g/day (up to 4 g may be used if necessary and tolerated). Side-effects include paresthesias, drowsiness, altered taste particularly for carbonated beverages. Rare but serious side-effects include Stevens–Johnson syndrome, renal stones, aplastic anemia, and allergic reaction
- Other diuretics may be used if acetazolamide is contraindicated or not tolerated, such as furosemide, triamterene, spironolactone
- Headache treatment
  - Topiramate (50–200 mg) may be useful for headache. Weight loss and carbonic anhydrase activity, which reduces CSF

production, may also lead to a reduction in intracranial pressure. Other medications such as divalproex sodium, amitriptyline, and verapamil, are less effective and may cause weight gain

- Indomethacin (25–75 mg three times daily) may be helpful for headache and may also lead to reduction in intracranial pressure
- Limit acute headache medications to no more than 2 days/week. Migraine specific medications (triptans/ergots) may be helpful, especially in those with a history of migraine

SURGERY

- Indications for surgery include:
  - Significant visual field loss at presentation
  - Deterioration in visual acuity or visual field despite aggressive medical therapy
- Optic nerve sheath fenestration (ONSF)
- Should be performed by experienced ophthalmologic surgeons. Creation of a fenestration (window) in the optic nerve sheath leads to immediate reduction in CSF pressure in the subarachnoid space surrounding the optic nerve
- Unilateral or bilateral simultaneous procedures
- Outcome
  - Visual field in ipsilateral eye improves in 75%
  - Visual acuity in contralateral eye improves in 50%
  - Headache improves in 60%
- Complications
  - Transient diplopia
  - Ocular discomfort
  - Tonic pupil

- Shunting
  - Headache improves in 95% but recurrence rate is almost 50% by 3 years
  - Shunt failure or low CSF pressure requiring revision occurs in at least 50%. Mean time to first revision is about 9 months. Shunt failure significantly more common in lumboperitoneal shunts (86%) compared with ventriculoperitoneal shunts (44%)
  - Complications include infection, low CSF pressure, Chiari malformation, radiculopathy
- Venous sinus stenting
  - Experience very limited
  - May be indicated in patients with medically unresponsive IIH and evidence of transverse venous sinus stenosis on MRV

■ Further reading

Brazis P. The surgical treatment of idiopathic pseudotumor cerebri (idiopathic intracranial hypertension). *Cephalalgia* 2008;**28**:1361–1373.

Friedman DI. Pseudotumor cerebri presenting as headache. *Exp Rev Neurother* 2008;**8**:397–407.

33

Intracranial neoplasm

■ Key points

- Headache is a common symptom in patients with brain tumors, occurring in 30%–60%
- Headache is rarely the sole clinical manifestation of a brain tumor (<10%)
- The headache of brain tumor is frequently nonspecific and may resemble tension-type headache, migraine headache, or other headache types
- Patients with headache "red flags" (Box 33.1) may need to be investigated for the presence of a secondary cause for their headache, such as a brain tumor

■ General overview

- Patients and physicians alike are often concerned that headaches may be a manifestation of an underlying brain tumor
- Headaches may occur secondary to primary brain tumors, metastatic brain tumor, and leptomeningeal malignancies
- Headache as the isolated presenting feature of an intracranial neoplasm is rare. Although headache is reported by 30%–60% of brain tumor patients at the time of diagnosis, in the majority of cases, there are clues in the patient's history, other symptoms, and physical exam findings supportive of the diagnosis

> **Box 33.1** Headache red flags
>
> - New-onset persistent or progressive headache
> - Change in headache characteristics as compared with prior headaches
> - Nausea and vomiting
> - Precipitated by changes in position or Valsalva
> - Awakens patient from sleep and/or worst upon awakening in the morning
> - Constitutional symptoms – weight loss, night sweats
> - Meningismus
> - History of neoplasm
> - Risk factors for neoplasm
> - Focal neurologic symptoms or signs
> - Papilledema

■ Clinical features

- Headache
  - More common in brain tumor patients with elevated intracranial pressure
  - Occurs as the isolated symptom of brain tumor in <10% of patients
  - Typical headache is bifrontal but worse on the side ipsilateral to the tumor
    - More likely to be diffuse in location if presence of elevated intracranial pressure/hydrocephalus
  - Most often a dull ache or pressure (may be mistaken for tension-type headache)
  - Usually moderate to severe in intensity
  - Most often intermittent

- May be associated with nausea and vomiting
- May worsen with bending over, Valsalva, other measures of increasing intracranial pressure and be worst upon awakening in the morning

- Seizures
  - More common with tumors involving the cortex
- Focal neurologic manifestations (vary widely according to the location of the tumor)
  - Weakness
  - Numbness
  - Speech change
  - Cognitive change
  - Ataxia
  - Visual change
  - Cranial nerve abnormalities

■ Diagnosis

- The diagnosis of headache secondary to brain tumor is dependent on a careful inquiry of worrisome features or red flags (see Box 33.1), physical and neurologic examination, and cerebral imaging when there is suspicion of tumor
- History
  - Headache red flags that increase suspicion for brain tumor (see Box 33.1)
  - Risk factors for neoplasm
    - Smoking
    - Family history
    - Known extracranial tumor
      - Tumors most likely to metastasize to the brain include lung, breast, kidney, melanoma
    - Exposure to ionizing radiation

- Physical exam
  - Neurologic exam
    - Cognitive impairment
    - Papilledema
    - Lateralizing neurologic abnormalities
      - Speech/language dysfunction
      - Weakness
      - Numbness
      - Visual field abnormalities
      - Gait instability
      - Limb or axial ataxia
      - Cranial nerve dysfunction
      - Asymmetric deep tendon reflexes
      - Babinski sign
- Imaging
  - MRI with gadolinium enhancement
    - Unless contraindicated, MRI with gadolinium is the initial imaging modality of choice as it is superior to CT with contrast in identifying and characterizing brain tumors
    - Tumor location, size, and characteristics
    - Surrounding edema
    - Compression of surrounding brain parenchyma
    - Hydrocephalus
    - Meningeal involvement
  - CT
    - Study of choice if MRI is contraindicated
    - Study of choice in the emergent setting if hemorrhage is suspected
    - Is superior to and complementary to MRI if suspicion of skull-based, clivus, or foramen magnum lesions

■ Treatment

- The treatment of headache secondary to a brain tumor is dependent on treatment of the underlying lesion and administration of analgesics
- Analgesics
  - ■ The majority of patients have at least partial response
    - ● Response to analgesics should not be considered evidence against the possibility of an underlying tumor
- Hydrocephalus
  - ■ Treatment of underlying hydrocephalus, if present
- Edema
  - ■ Corticosteroids for reduction of surrounding edema, if present
- Tumor
  - ■ Treatment of underlying tumor

■ Further reading

Cha S. Update on brain tumor imaging. *Curr Neurol Neurosci Rep* 2005;**5**:169–177.

Forsyth PA, Posner JB. Headaches in patients with brain tumors: a study of 111 patients. *Neurology* 1993;**43**:1678–1683.

Norden AD, Wen PY, Kesari S. Brain metastases. *Curr Opin Neurol* 2005;**18**:654–661.

Vazquez-Barquero A, Ibanez FJ, Izaquierdo JM, *et al.* Isolated headache as the presenting clinical manifestation of intracranial tumors: a prospective study. *Cephalalgia* 1994;**14**:270–272.

Wrensch M, Minn Y, *et al.* Epidemiology of primary brain tumors: current concepts and review of the literature. *Neuro-oncology* 2002;**4**:278–299.

34

Sinus headache

■ Key points

- Headache and/or facial pain are common manifestations of acute rhinosinusitis
- A diagnosis of sinus headache requires a temporal relationship between the onset of acute rhinosinusitis (fevers, purulent drainage, etc.) and the onset of headache
- It is likely that the majority of patients with self-diagnosed "sinus headaches" really have migraine headache
- Chronic sinusitis is not formally recognized as a cause of headache
- Since imaging findings correlate poorly with patient symptoms, clinical manifestations must be present in order to diagnose acute rhinosinusitis and rhinosinusitis headache

■ General overview

- Since both headaches and sinus disease are common conditions, their simultaneous presence does not stipulate a diagnosis of sinus headache
- However, headache or facial pain can occur with acute sinusitis
- The sinuses and nasal mucosa are innervated by branches of the trigeminal nerve, the same nerve responsible for facial and head pain

- Although imaging of the sinuses can be helpful in the evaluation of patients with sinus disease and contribute to the diagnoses of sinusitis and sinus headache, these diagnoses require the presence of clinical symptoms

■ Clinical features

- Headaches
  - Frontal in location
  - Usually bilateral and periorbital
  - Pressurelike and dull
  - Worse in the morning with improvement as the day progresses
  - Associated with pain in the face, ears, or teeth
    - May worsen with bending forward
  - Pain may vary with changes in atmospheric pressure
  - Must begin at the same time as the sinusitis
  - Must resolve within 7 days of successful treatment of the sinusitis
- Fever
- Purulent nasal discharge
- Nasal congestion
- Hyposmia/anosmia
- Halitosis
- Ear pain/fullness

■ Diagnosis

- The International Headache Society diagnostic criteria for headache associated with acute rhinosinusitis are listed in Box 34.1
- The American Academy of Otolaryngology – Head and Neck Surgery (AAO-HNS) diagnostic criteria for rhinosinusitis are listed in Box 34.2

Box 34.1 Headache associated with acute rhinosinusitis –
International Headache Society diagnostic criteria

A. Frontal headache accompanied by pain in one or more
   regions of the face, ears or teeth and fulfilling criteria C and D

B. Clinical (purulence in the nasal cavity, nasal obstruction,
   hyposmia, anosmia, and/or fever), nasal endoscopic, CT and/
   or MRI and/or laboratory evidence of acute or acute-on-
   chronic rhinosinusitis

C. Headache and/or facial pain develop simultaneously with
   onset or acute exacerbation of rhinosinusitis

D. Headache and/or facial pain resolve within 7 days after
   remission or successful treatment of acute or acute-on-
   chronic rhinosinusitis

- Physical exam
  - Fever
  - Tenderness to percussion/palpation over the affected
    sinuses
  - Transillumination
  - Nasal endoscopy
- Laboratory evaluation
  - May not be necessary in cases of uncomplicated (neither
    intracranial nor orbital involvement is suspected),
    community-acquired sinusitis
  - Complete blood count
  - Sinus aspirate culture
    - Gold-standard for the diagnosis of sinusitis
- Imaging
  - Imaging is not necessary in uncomplicated cases of sinusitis in
    which the diagnosis can be made on clinical grounds

Box 34.2 Rhinosinusitis – AAO-HNS diagnostic criteria

Diagnosis requires ≥2 major factors or ≥1 major factor and ≥2 minor factors

Major factors:

- Purulence in nasal cavity
- Facial pain/pressure/congestion/fullness
- Nasal obstruction/blockage/discharge/purulence
- Fever (acute rhinosinusitis only)
- Hyposmia/anosmia

Minor factors:

- Headache
- Fever (all nonacute)
- Halitosis
- Fatigue
- Dental pain
- Cough
- Ear pain/fullness

- CT sinus (Fig. 34.1)
  - Air–fluid levels
  - Sinus opacification
  - Mucosal thickening
  - Poor correlation between facial and/or head pain and CT sinus findings
- MRI
  - Useful if intracranial spread of infection is suspected

■ Treatment

- The treatment of sinus headache depends on successful treatment of the underlying sinusitis

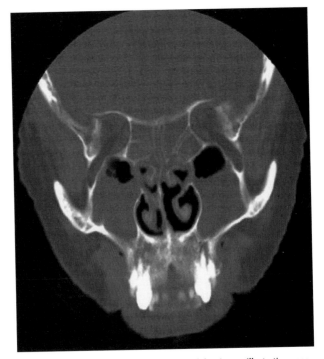

Fig. 34.1 Coronal computed tomography scan of the sinuses illustrating near complete impaction of the maxillary sinuses in a patient with acute bilateral maxillary sinusitis and maxillary facial and frontal head pain.

■ Further reading

Cady RK, Dodick DW, Levine HL, *et al*. Sinus headache: a neurology, otolaryngology, allergy, and primary care consensus on diagnosis and treatment. *Mayo Clin Proc* 2005; **80**:908–916.

Cady RK, Schreiber CP. Sinus headache or migraine? Considerations in making a differential diagnosis. *Neurology* 2002;**58**:S10–S14.

Lanza DC, Kennedy DW. Adult rhinosinusitis defined. *Otolaryngol Head Neck Surg* 1997;**117**:S1–S7.

Mudgil SP, Wise SW, Hopper KD, *et al.* Correlation between presumed sinusitis-induced pain and paranasal sinus computed tomographic findings. *Ann Allergy Asthma Immunol* 2002;**88**:223–226.

35

Medication-overuse headache

■ Key point

- Use of simple analgesics (i.e., ibuprofen) or any combination of acute headache medications ≥15 days per month *or* use of combination analgesics (containing caffeine, codeine, or barbiturates), opioids, ergotamine, or triptans ≥10 days per month can "transform" episodic headaches into a near-daily or daily pattern

■ General overview

- Medication-overuse headache (MOH) refers to the generation, perpetuation, or maintenance of chronic head pain in headache sufferers, caused by the frequent and excessive use of immediate-relief (symptomatic) medications
- MOH was previously called "rebound headache" and "drug-induced headache."
- The criteria for overuse are specific for the type of medication being overused:
  - Any combination of acute/symptomatic medications on ≥15 days per month
  - Simple analgesics on ≥15 days per month
  - Opioid-containing analgesics on ≥10 days per month

- Combination medication containing caffeine or barbiturates or codeine on ≥10 days per month
- Triptans or ergotamine on ≥10 days per month
- The prevalence of MOH in the general population is approximately 1.5%
- The prevalence is higher in women than in men (3.5:1)
- In tertiary headache centers in the United States, 50%–80% of patients meet the criteria for MOH
- MOH is important to recognize because overusing medications can perpetuate and chronify the underlying headache condition, and, importantly, may lead to dose-related toxicity from the overused medication
- Clinical observation and expert opinion suggest that MOH may "neutralize" the effectiveness of traditional prophylactic agents; however, this has not been definitively proven in clinical trials

■ Clinical features

- Headache
  - The revised ICHD-2 diagnostic criteria for MOH state that there are no particular headache characteristics that are necessary or sufficient to make a diagnosis of MOH
  - Individuals with MOH typically experience the following:
    - The frequency of the headaches increases insidiously over time
    - Patients often awake in the early morning with headache (even though this was not a feature of their original headache)
    - A proportion of individual headache attacks may become nondescript (losing their characteristic migrainous or autonomic features and phenotypically resembling tension-type headache)

- The threshold for stress or exertion to precipitate headaches is frequently lowered
- Escalating doses of symptomatic medications are required
- Headaches recur within a predictable time period after the last consumption of symptomatic medication (due to rebound or withdrawal phenomenon)
- Associated features
  - Depending on the characteristics of the overused medication, the individual may experience concentration difficulties, forgetfulness, restlessness, anxiety, irritability, nausea, and other cognitive, psychological, and gastrointestinal symptoms

■ Diagnosis

- The diagnosis of medication overuse headache is based on operational diagnostic criteria (see Box 35.1)
- The differential diagnosis of MOH includes chronic migraine (see Chapter 25), chronic tension-type headache [CTTH] Chapter 26), new daily persistent headache (see Chapter 28) and other secondary headache disorders
- At initial presentation, the individual who is overusing acute headache medication in the setting of a preexisting primary headache disorder (i.e., migraine or tension-type headache) can be diagnosed only with *probable* medication overuse headache and *probable* chronic migraine or *probable* chronic tension-type headache
- The only way to definitively determine whether the chronic daily headache (CDH) is attributable to MOH or to the underlying primary or secondary headache disorder is to completely withdraw the offending overused acute headache medication for 2 months. If after 2 months the headache has disappeared or

Box 35.1 Medication-overuse headache – International Headache Society revised diagnostic criteria

8.2 Medication-overuse headache

Diagnostic criteria:

A. Headache present on ≥15 days/month fulfilling criteria C and D
B. Regular overuse for >3 months of one or more drugs that can be taken for acute and/or symptomatic treatment of headache
C. Headache has developed or markedly worsened during medication overuse
D. Headache resolves or reverts to its previous pattern within 2 months after discontinuation of overused medication

8.2.1 Ergotamine-overuse headache

Diagnostic criteria:

A. Headache fulfilling criteria A, C and D for 8.2 *Medication-overuse headache*
B. Ergotamine intake on ≥10 days/month on a regular basis for >3 months

8.2.2 Triptan-overuse headache

Diagnostic criteria:

A. Headache fulfilling criteria A, C and D for 8.2 *Medication-overuse headache*
B. Triptan intake (any formulation) on ≥10 days/month on a regular basis for >3 months

8.2.3 Analgesic-overuse headache

Diagnostic criteria

A. Headache fulfilling criteria A, C and D for 8.2 *Medication-overuse headache*
B. Intake of simple analgesics on ≥15 days/month on a regular basis for >3 months

8.2.4 Opioid-overuse headache

Diagnostic criteria:

A. Headache fulfilling criteria A, C and D for 8.2 *Medication-overuse headache*

B. Opioid intake on ≥10 days/month on a regular basis for >3 months

Comment:
Prospective studies indicate that patients overusing opioids have the highest relapse rate after withdrawal treatment.

8.2.5 Combination analgesic-overuse headache

Diagnostic criteria:

A. Headache fulfilling criteria A, C and D for 8.2 *Medication-overuse headache*

B. Intake of combination analgesic medications on ≥10 days/month on a regular basis for >3 months

8.2.6 Medication-overuse headache attributed to combination of acute medications

Diagnostic criteria:

A. Headache fulfilling criteria A, C and D for 8.2 *Medication-overuse headache*

B. Intake of any combination of ergotamine, triptans, analgesics and/or opioids on ≥10 days/month on a regular basis for >3 months without overuse of any single class alone

8.2.7 Headache attributed to other medication overuse

Diagnostic criteria:

A. Headache fulfilling criteria A, C and D for 8.2 *Medication-overuse headache*

B. Regular overuse for >3 months of a medication other than those described above

8.2.8 Probable medication-overuse headache

Diagnostic criteria

A. Headache fulfilling criteria A and C for 8.2 *Medication-overuse headache*

B. Medication overuse fulfilling criterion B for any one of the subforms 8.2.1–8.2.7

C. One or other of the following:
1. overused medication has not yet been withdrawn
2. medication overuse has ceased within the last 2 months but headache has not so far resolved or reverted to its previous pattern

significantly improved, the headache can be appropriately labeled as MOH. In contrast, if after 2 months medication withdrawal the headache remains unchanged, the affected individual can be appropriately considered to have a chronic form of the underlying headache disorder (i.e., chronic migraine or CTTH)

■ Pathophysiology

- The underlying pathophysiology of MOH remains unclear; however, proposed mechanisms include:
  - Psychotropic effects of, and corresponding withdrawal effects from, caffeine, codeine, or barbiturates
  - Downregulation of central inhibitory pathways, resulting in a reduction of descending inhibitory modulation and the facilitation of trigeminal nociception
  - Paradoxical pronociceptive effects, whereby frequent opioid administration leads to increased activity of pain facilitation

cells (ON-cells) arising in the rostral ventromedial medulla, an area essential to the integration of nociceptive processing and descending pain modulation

- Migraineurs may have an underlying genetic susceptibility to MOH, considering that patients with other painful disorders but no headaches who require daily analgesics do not develop CDH. Interestingly, in a study of 110 patients using daily analgesics for rheumatologic disorders, an increased risk of developing CDH occurred only in "susceptible" individuals with a preexisting history of episodic migraine

■ Treatment

- No blinded, placebo-controlled, medication-withdrawal trials in patients with CDH suspected of having MOH have been done. Because of ethical concerns and pragmatic issues, it is unlikely that these trials will ever be performed
- The following steps reflect our approach to dealing with MOH.
  1. Education – patients must be educated about their headaches and medication overuse so they can assume an active role in the treatment process
  2. Lifestyle modifications – establish a regular and appropriate sleep pattern, avoid skipping meals, initiate a regular exercise program, and eliminate caffeine consumption
  3. Withdrawal of overused medications – overused medications can often be abruptly discontinued. They are tapered when the possibility of tolerance, habituation and dependence, exists
     - Abrupt discontinuation – this can be done for simple analgesics, ergotamines, triptans and most combined analgesics

- Taper – withdrawal from opioids and/or barbiturates must be slow rather than abrupt. To alleviate potential side-effects from barbiturate withdrawal, a long-acting barbiturate alternative (i.e., phenobarbital) may be substituted and tapered
- Acute headache management
  - Withdrawal symptoms typically last for 2–10 days. Symptomatic agents in limited doses (from drug classes other than those which they are overusing) should be provided to alleviate withdrawal symptoms (headache, nausea, vomiting, arterial hypotension, tachycardia, sleep disturbances, restlessness, and nervousness)
  - Options include long-acting NSAIDs, dihydroergotamine ([DHE] 1 mg intranasal, subcutaneously, or intramuscularly), triptans, or an oral prednisone taper
  - For patients requiring more aggressive treatment, several strategies have been advocated: intravenous or daily subcutaneous DHE, intravenous methylprednisolone, intravenous neuroleptics, and intravenous divalproex sodium or some combination thereof
  - After initial detoxification, acute medications (i.e., NSAIDs or triptans) are provided in limited doses to treat episodic migraine attacks
4. Prophylactic therapy – there is no solid evidence on which to base prophylactic therapy decisions in these patients; however, reasonable options include: antidepressants (e.g., amitriptyline), anticonvulsants (i.e., topiramate, gabapentin and divalproex sodium), neurotoxins (i.e., botulinum toxin), and possibly antispasticity agents (i.e. tizanidine)
5. Bio-behavioral therapy – relaxation therapy, biofeedback, stress-management, and cognitive-behavioral therapy are often helpful to allow patients to achieve an internal locus of control

6. Comorbid disorders – comorbid depression and/or anxiety should be addressed concurrently (note that some patients are depressed *because* of their daily headache)

7. Follow-up – patients should be given support with close follow-up and educated about realistic expectations (i.e., individuals who overuse medications need to realize that during the withdrawal phase they may feel worse before they feel better)

8. Referral – as management of these patients is often time-consuming and difficult, early referral to a neurologist and/or a headache clinic is justified

■ Outcome

- There is a wide range in the reported relapse rates following withdrawal of overused acute headache medications. The relapse rates vary with the location of withdrawal (inpatient versus outpatient), the strategies utilized to withdrawal the patient (cold-turkey, parenteral medication protocol such as intravenous DHE), the type of medication overused, and the length of follow-up
- Prospective studies indicate that patients overusing opioids have the highest relapse rate after withdrawal treatment

■ Further reading

Boes CH, Capobianco DJ. Chronic migraine and medication-overuse headache through the ages. *Cephalalgia* 2005;**25**:378–390.

Boes CJ, Black DF, Dodick DW. Pathophysiology and management of transformed migraine and medication overuse headache. *Semin Neurol* 2006;**26**:232–241.

Diener HC, Limmroth V. Medication-overuse headache: a worldwide problem. *Lancet Neurol* 2004;**3**:475–483.

Dodick D, Freitag F. Evidence-based understanding of medication-overuse headache: clinical implications. *Headache* 2006;**46**(Suppl 4):S202–S211.

Dowson AJ, Dodick DW, Limmroth V. Medication overuse headache in patients with primary headache disorders: epidemiology, management and pathogenesis. *CNS Drugs* 2005;**19**:483–497.

Lake AE, 3rd. Medication overuse headache: biobehavioral issues and solutions. *Headache* 2006;**46**(Suppl 3):S88–S97.

Meskunas CA, Tepper SJ, Rapoport AM, *et al.* Medications associated with probable medication overuse headache reported in a tertiary care headache center over a 15-year period. *Headache* 2006;**46**:766–772.

Silberstein SD, Olesen J, Bousser MG, *et al.* International Classification of Headache Disorders, 2nd Edition (ICHD-II) – revision of 8.2 Medication Overuse Headache. *Cephalalgia* 2005;**25**:460–465.

Zeeberg P, Olesen J, Jensen R. Discontinuation of medication overuse in headache patients: recovery of therapeutic responsiveness. *Cephalalgia* 2006;**26**:1192–1198.

Zeeberg P, Olesen J, Jensen R. Probable medication-overuse headache: the effect of a 2-month drug-free period. *Neurology* 2006;**66**:1894–1898.

36

Post-traumatic headache

■ Key points

- Headache is one of many symptoms that may occur after head injury
- Headache is the most common symptom of the post-traumatic syndrome
- Outcome is usually the same whether or not litigation is involved

■ General overview

- Post-traumatic headache (PTH) is a spectrum of acute to chronic headache patterns that are frequently accompanied by other symptoms following mild to severe head injury
- Tension headache is most common pattern of PTH
- PTH needs careful assessment and expert management

■ Clinical features (Boxes 36.1, 36.2, 36.3, and 36.4)

- Headache
  - The nature of the headache is nonspecific, but tends to resemble tension-type headache in 80% of cases; migraine or rarely cluster can be the clinical presentation of PTH

Box 36.1 Acute posttraumatic headache attributed to moderate to severe head injury – International Headache Society diagnostic criteria

A. Headache, no typical characteristics known, fulfilling criteria C and D

B. Head trauma with at least one of the following:
   1. loss of consciousness for >30 minutes
   2. Glasgow Coma Scale (GCS) <13
   3. post-traumatic amnesia for >48 hours
   4. imaging demonstration of a traumatic brain lesion (cerebral haematoma, intracerebral and/or subarachnoid haemorrhage, brain contusion and/or skull fracture)

C. Headache develops within 7 days after head trauma or after regaining consciousness following head trauma

D. One or other of the following:
   1. headache resolves within 3 months after head trauma
   2. headache persists but 3 months have not yet passed since head trauma

- Other accompanying symptoms may include:
  - Dizziness
  - Difficulty with concentration
  - Nervousness
  - Personality changes
  - Insomnia
- Risk factor for developing PTH
  - Women have higher risk for PTH
  - Paradoxically, headache may be less frequent in more severe head injury
  - PTH is more common in patients with pre-existing primary headaches

Box 36.2 Acute posttraumatic headache attributed to mild head injury – International Headache Society diagnostic criteria

A. Headache, no typical characteristics known, fulfilling criteria C and D

B. Head trauma with all the following:
  1. either no loss of consciousness, or loss of consciousness of <30 minutes' duration
  2. Glasgow Coma Scale (GCS) ≥13
  3. symptoms and/or signs diagnostic of concussion

C. Headache develops within 7 days after head trauma

D. One or other of the following:
  1. headache resolves within 3 months after head trauma
  2. headache persists but 3 months have not yet passed since head trauma

Box 36.3 Chronic posttraumatic headache attributed to moderate to severe head injury – International Headache Society diagnostic criteria

A. Headache, no typical characteristics known, fulfilling criteria C and D

B. Head trauma with at least one of the following:
  1. loss of consciousness for >30 minutes
  2. Glasgow Coma Scale (GCS) <13
  3. post-traumatic amnesia for >48 hours
  4. imaging demonstration of a traumatic brain lesion (cerebral haematoma, intracerebral and/or subarachnoid haemorrhage, brain contusion and/or skull fracture)

C. Headache develops within 7 days after head trauma or after regaining consciousness following head trauma

D. Headache persists for >3 months after head trauma

Box 36.4 Chronic posttraumatic headache attributed to mild head injury – International Headache Society diagnostic criteria

A. Headache, no typical characteristics known, fulfilling criteria C and D

B. Head trauma with all the following:
   1. either no loss of consciousness, or loss of consciousness of <30 minutes' duration
   2. Glasgow Coma Scale (GCS) ≥13
   3. symptoms and/or signs diagnostic of concussion

C. Headache develops within 7 days after head trauma

D. Headache persists for >3 months after head trauma

- Mechanical factors including head position: inclined or rotated position makes PTH less likely
- With increasing age, there is less rapid and complete recovery

■ Diagnosis

- Physical exam
  - Neurologic exam
    - If focal neurologic signs are present further investigations are needed to rule out more serious sequelae of trauma
  - Musculoskeletal exam
    - Tenderness with palpation of the skull (including digital pressure in the region of the greater occipital nerves) and neck structures can demonstrate trigger points
- Imaging
  - Usually not contributory but can rule out secondary or other serious causes of headache including subdural or epidural hematoma

- CT
  - Good for visualizing bone structure and fractures of skull
  - Useful in the emergent setting for assessment of intracranial hemorrhage
- MRI
  - Better anatomic definition of head and neck structures, as well as the brain and spinal cord
  - Most are normal, however some white matter changes have been noted.

Treatment

- Symptomatic
  - Analgesics
  - Migraine therapies for those with migraine symptoms and cluster treatments for cluster symptoms
- Prevention
  - Amitriptyline
    - Use low dosages initially to avoid side-effects
    - Has added benefit of treating comorbid affective disorders if present
  - Use migraine prophylactic medications for those with a migraine pattern of headache, tension-type medications for those with tension-type headache symptoms, and cluster treatments for those with a cluster pattern
  - Nonpharmacologic therapy is important
    - Behavioral therapies, including general psychological support

Outcome

- Depends on multiple factors as per diagnostic criteria
- Litigation might appear important, but outcome is not different in terms of time to improvement, types of headache, and

response to migraine medications in patients who pursue litigation and those who do not. Also symptoms do not usually resolve with litigation settlement

- Causal relationship between headache and mild trauma is difficult to establish
- Up to ⅓ of patients do not return to work after mild head injury

■ Further reading

Evans RW. Post-traumatic headaches. *Neurol Clin* 2004;**22**:237–249.

Headache Classification Subcommittee of the International Headache Society. The International Classification Headache Disorders, 2nd edn. *Cephalalgia* 2004;**24**(Suppl 1): 9–160.

Young W, Packard RC, Ramadan N. Headache associated with head trauma. In: Siberstein SD, Lipton RB, Dalessio DJ, eds. *Wolff's Headache and Other Head Pain*. Oxford: Oxford University Press, 2001: 325–348.

37

Cervicogenic headache

■ Key points

- The term "cervicogenic headache" refers to headaches generated by sources in the cervical region
- Clinical, laboratory, and/or imaging evidence of an abnormality of the upper cervical spine or in the soft tissues of the neck is necessary for the diagnosis of cervicogenic headache
- Formal diagnosis requires resolution of pain following blockade of the cervical nerves or their branches

■ General overview

- Cervicogenic headaches are caused by abnormalities of the cervical spine or in the soft tissues of the neck
- Due to physiological continuity between the upper cervical spinal cord and the trigeminal nerve, structures innervated by C1–C3 nerves may be a source of cervicogenic headache
- Cervical spine structures caudal to C3 may also cause cervicogenic headache, although this relationship is less clear
- Since cervical pain is a common feature of many headache types, the presence of such pain alone does not indicate a diagnosis of cervicogenic headache

■ Clinical features

- Headache
  - Predominantly unilateral
    - May be felt bilaterally when pain is severe
  - Moderate to severe in severity
  - Nonthrobbing, nonlancinating
  - Starts in the neck and radiates forward to the occipital, parietal, temporal, frontal, and ocular regions in a C-shaped pattern
  - Pain may be episodic or continuous with fluctuating severity
  - Attack-related phenomena include:
    - Autonomic symptoms and signs (conjunctival injection, lacrimation, eyelid edema, rhinorrhea, nasal congestion)
    - Nausea/vomiting
    - Photophobia
    - Phonophobia
    - Ipsilateral edema in the periorbital region
    - Ipsilateral blurred vision
    - Dizziness
    - Discomfort in the throat/swallowing difficulties
- Cervical features
  - Pain involves the neck with radiation to the posterior and then anterior regions of the head
  - Movements of the neck or sustained head posture may precipitate head pain
  - External pressure on the occiput/subocciput or upper neck may precipitate head pain
  - Restricted range of motion of the neck
- Additional features
  - May have ipsilateral shoulder and arm pain

■ Diagnosis

- Based on: clinical features, evidence for a source of pain in the neck, and efficacy of diagnostic blockades (Box 37.1)
- Physical exam
  - Abnormal neck posture
  - Decrease in the range of motion of the neck
  - Head pain is triggered by neck movements and/or pressure on the occiput/subocciput or upper part of the neck
  - Muscular trigger points

Box 37.1 Cervicogenic headache – International Headache Society diagnostic criteria

A. Pain, referred from a source in the neck and perceived in one or more regions of the head and/or face, fulfilling criteria C and D

B. Clinical, laboratory and/or imaging evidence of a disorder or lesion within the cervical spine or soft tissues of the neck known to be, or generally accepted as, a valid cause of headache

C. Evidence that the pain can be attributed to the neck disorder or lesion based on at least one of the following:
  1. demonstration of clinical signs that implicate a source of pain in the neck
  2. abolition of headache following diagnostic blockade of a cervical structure or its nerve supply using placebo or other adequate controls

D. Pain resolves within 3 months after successful treatment of the causative disorder or lesion

- Imaging
  - May provide evidence for the diagnosis
    - Imaging abnormalities of the cervical spine in isolation of appropriate symptoms, physical exam findings, and/or response to appropriate nerve blocks cannot be diagnostic for cervicogenic headache
  - May include cervical spine radiographs, MRI, and/or CT myelography
- Diagnostic nerve blockade
  - May include the following locations:
    - Greater occipital nerve
    - Lesser occipital nerve
    - Cervical segmental nerves (first three cervical spinal nerves)
    - Cervical facet joints (zygapophyseal joints) (C2–C3, C3–C4)
  - According to the International Headache Society diagnostic criteria (Box 37.1), a placebo control must be used; however, in clinical (non-research) scenarios, this may be impractical

■ Treatment

- Combined approach using medications, physical therapy, anesthetic, and, occasionally, surgical intervention
- The initial approach generally includes medication and/or anesthetic blockade in conjunction with physical therapy
  - If this approach is ineffective, neurolytic procedures may be indicated
  - If neurolytic procedures are ineffective, cervical epidural steroid injections or surgical intervention may be indicated

- Medications (none are approved by the United States Food and Drug Administration for cervicogenic headache)
  - Includes many of the drugs used to treat the primary headache disorders:
    - Antiepileptics
    - Antidepressants
    - NSAIDs
    - Muscle relaxants
- Physical therapy
  - May include the use of transcutaneous electrical nerve stimulation (TENS)
- Anesthetic blockade
  - Same locations as discussed under "Diagnostic nerve blockade"
- Neurolytic procedures
  - If anesthetic blockades are effective but of inadequate duration, radiofrequency ablation or other lytic procedures may be considered
- Cervical epidural steroid injections
  - May be considered in those patients with inadequate response to anesthetic blocks and neurolytic procedures
- Surgical procedures
  - Nerve destruction – may result in postoperative pain syndrome (anesthesia dolorosa)
  - Spinal nerve stimulation
  - Occipital nerve stimulation

■ Further reading

Bartsch T, Goadsby PJ. Anatomy and physiology of pain referral patterns in primary and cervicogenic headache disorders. *Headache Curr* 2005;**2**:42–48.

Biondi DM. Cervicogenic headache: a review of diagnostic and treatment strategies. *J Am Osteopath Assoc* 2005;**105** (Suppl 2):S16–S22.

Bogduk N. Distinguishing primary headache disorders from cervicogenic headache: clinical and therapeutic implications. *Headache Curr* 2005;**2**:27–36.

Fredriksen TA, Hovdal H, Sjaastad O. "Cervicogenic headache": clinical manifestation. *Cephalalgia* 1987;**7**:147–160.

Silverman SB. Cervicogenic headache: interventional, anesthetic, and ablative treatment. *Curr Pain Headache Rep* 2002;**6**:308–314.

38

Occipital neuralgia

■ Key points

- Neuralgic pain involving the territories of the lesser or greater occipital nerves
- Tenderness to palpation over the affected nerves
- Pain temporarily improves or resolves after anesthetic blockade of the affected nerves

■ General overview

- The occipital nerve is derived from the second cervical nerve root
- The occipital nerve is responsible for sensation to the posterior head, portions of the neck, and portions of the face (peri-/retro-orbital)
- Onset preceded by minor trauma to the head or neck in about ¼ of patients
  - Mild head trauma
  - Cervical strain from motor vehicle accident or fall
- More common in women
- Most patients with occipital neuralgia do not have a demonstrable lesion accounting for the pain
  - Exceptions include neuromas and upper cervical root compression from spondylosis or ligamentous hypertrophy
- Chronic muscle tension and spasm may cause irritation of the nerves

Clinical features

- Headache
  - Brief, lancinating, sharp, paroxysmal pain in the posterior region(s) of the head
    - Unilateral or bilateral
    - May radiate anteriorly to the ipsilateral temporal, frontal, and retro-orbital regions, and caudally to the ipsilateral cervical regions
    - Lasts for several seconds
    - May occur several times per day
  - Some patients have an underlying continuous, dull, aching pain in the same distribution as the neuralgic pains
  - May be exacerbated by neck flexion
- Ocular symptoms
  - Visual blurring
  - Ocular pain
  - Lacrimation
- Tinnitus
- Dizziness/vertigo
- Nausea
- Scalp paresthesias
- Photophobia
- Nasal congestion

Diagnosis (Box 38.1)

- Physical exam
  - Tenderness over the affected nerve (Tinel sign)
    - Lesser occipital nerve – palpate about 3 cm superior and medial to the mastoid process

> **Box 38.1 Occipital neuralgia – International Headache Society diagnostic criteria**
>
> A. Paroxysmal stabbing pain, with or without persistent aching between paroxysms, in the distribution(s) of the greater, lesser and/or third occipital nerves
> B. Tenderness over the affected nerve
> C. Pain is eased temporarily by local anesthetic block of the nerve

- Greater occipital nerve – palpate over the occipital protuberance
  - Neck tenderness
  - Abnormal sensation in the C2 dermatome
- Imaging
  - Cervical spine
    - If the pain is suspected to have a cervical origin, imaging of the cervical spine is indicated
  - Brain and/or vertebrobasilar arteries
    - Consider if posterior head pain is accompanied by features atypical for occipital neuralgia
    - Presence of neurological deficits other than abnormal sensation in the territory of the affected nerve

■ Treatment

- Occipital nerve blockade
  - Anesthetic (e.g., bupivacaine) plus/minus steroid
  - Provides relief from pain and associated symptoms
    - Effects last days to months
    - If pain returns it is often less severe
- Physical therapy
- Analgesics – NSAIDs

- Preventive medications:
  - Gabapentin
  - Tricyclic antidepressants
  - Baclofen
  - Carbamazepine
  - Pregabalin
- Transcutaneous electrical nerve stimulation (TENS)
- Occipital nerve stimulation
  - Experimental approach
  - Reserved for patients who are nonresponsive to more conventional therapies
- Destructive procedures
  - Occasionally performed in patients nonresponsive to more conservative treatments
  - Successful in only a minority
  - May result in permanent pain or worsening of pain from denervation dysesthesia
  - Options include:
    - Chemical, thermal, or surgical ablation
    - Nerve sectioning of the peripheral nerve in the scalp or at the upper cervical dorsal root exit zone
    - Neurolysis
    - Foraminal decompression of C2 roots
    - C2 ganglionectomy

■ Further reading

Chouret EE. The greater occipital neuralgia headache. *Headache* 1967;**7**:33–34.

Kuhn WF, Kuhn SC, Gilberstadt H. Occipital neuralgias: clinical recognition of a complicated headache. A case series and literature review. *J Orofac Pain* 1997;**11**:158–165.

Sjaastad O, Fredrikson TA, Stolt-Nielsen A. Cervicogenic headache, C2 rhizopathy, and occipital neuralgia: a connection? *Cephalalgia* 1986;**6**:189–195.

Ward JB. Greater occipital nerve block. *Semin Neurol* 2003;**1**:59–61.

Weiner RL, Reed KL. Peripheral neurostimulation for control of intractable occipital neuralgia. *Neuromodulation* 1999;**2**:217–221.

39

Hypnic headache

■ Key points

- Headache occurs exclusively during nocturnal sleep (often at the same time each night) and during naps
- Headache occurs predominantly in older age group (mean age 64 years)
- Headache lasts 10–180 minutes; patients often need to sit or stand up for relief
- Attacks occur in both REM and NREM sleep; polysomnography required to exclude sleep-related breathing disorder and nocturnal hypertension
- Imaging is required to exclude pituitary, parasellar, or other intracranial lesion
- Caffeine, lithium carbonate, indomethacin, and melatonin are treatments of first choice

■ General overview

- Hypnic headache is a rare (0.07%) headache disorder occurring exclusively during sleep and primarily in older adults (>50 years), though patients as young as 9 years have been described
- Distinguished from cluster headache by the lack of cranial autonomic symptoms and the less than excruciating intensity

- Distinguished from migraine based on its occurrence only during sleep, its short duration and typical lack of migraine associated symptoms (e.g. photophobia, phonophobia)
- Attacks occur on at least 15 nights per month, at least one attack per night, often at the same time each night ("alarm clock headache"); 60% of patients report the first attack between 0100 and 0300 hours. Up to six attacks per night can occur
- Disorders that can mimic hypnic headache include obstructive sleep apnea, nocturnal hypertension, pituitary and other intracranial lesions

■ Clinical features

- Headache
  - Occurs on at least 15 nights per month; severe in ⅓, and mild-moderate in ⅔ of patients
  - Often occurs at or near the same time each night (commonly between 2 and 4 hours after falling asleep), may reoccur throughout the night, and during daytime naps
  - Lasts for 10–180 minutes
  - Throbbing in ⅓, dull/aching in ⅔, frontotemporal in 40%, and unilateral in ⅓
  - Improves on sitting, lying inclined, or on standing
- Associated symptoms
  - Mild nausea (<20%)
  - Photophobia, phonophobia, or both (in 7%)
  - Cranial autonomic symptoms rare

■ Diagnosis

- Clinical diagnosis based on characteristic clinical features
- Hypnic headache is distinguished from cluster headache and trigeminal autonomic cephalalgias, which also may have a

nocturnal predominance, by the lack of attacks during periods of wakefulness, lack of cranial autonomic features, and the milder nature of the pain. Attacks are more often bilateral or diffuse as opposed to cluster headache, which is side-locked with pain maximal in the periorbital region

- Overnight polysomnography is indicated to exclude obstructive sleep apnea and nocturnal hypertension. Most attacks (75%) occur during REM sleep
- Brain MRI is necessary to rule out intracranial lesions including pituitary and posterior fossa lesions, which cannot be reliably excluded with CT

TREATMENT

- Caffeine in the form of a cup of coffee or caffeine tablet (60–200 mg) may, paradoxically, be effective without significant sleep disruption
- Melatonin 3–12 mg prior to bedtime
- Indomethacin 25–75 mg prior to bedtime
- Lithium carbonate 300–600 mg

Other treatments with anecdotal success include botulinum neurotoxin type A, topiramate, pregabalin, triptans, and sedative-hypnotics, including diphenhydramine, doxylamine, and eszopiclone

■ Further reading

Evers S, Goadsby PJ. Hypnic headache: clinical features, pathophysiology, and treatment. *Neurology* 2003;**60**:905–909.

Liang JF, Fuh JL, Yu HY, *et al.* Clinical features, polysomnography and outcome in patients with hypnic headache. *Cephalalgia* 2008;**28**:209–215.

Index

Note: page numbers in *italics* refer to figures, tables